Healthy Hair,

Happy Body

By Simone Thomas

W: www.simonethomaswellness.com

ISBN: 978-1-7399121-0-9

First published in 2021

Copyright © 2021 Simone Thomas

Disclaimer

Although the author and publisher have made every effort to ensure that the information in this book was correct at press time, the author and publisher do not assume and hereby disclaim any liability to any party for any loss, damage, or disruption caused by errors or omissions, whether such errors or omissions result from negligence, accident, or any other cause. This book is not intended as a substitute for the advice of medical professionals, including mental health professionals. The reader should regularly consult a health professional in matters relating to his/her health, and particularly with respect to any symptoms that may require diagnosis, medical or psychological attention.

"Truly inspiring, Simone empowers you to improve your health and shares her knowledge with honesty and humour.

I have been lucky enough to have Simone on my hair loss journey, this book will guide you to a happier body and healthy hair...I am living proof!"

Paula Dale

"Simone was brilliant. I suffered with postnatal hair loss, and her team helped my hair grow back."

Georgie Culley

"Simone is a genuinely lovely and warm person, and the story of how she came to create her incredible supplements is truly emotional and uplifting. You might not be able to bottle up happiness, but she has found a way to bottle up healthier hair, skin and nails! From my own experience, I couldn't believe how much of a difference using her products made in a relatively short amount of time. I am sure that her biotin tablets healed a split nail that had been dogging me for years. I can't stop recommending her products to everyone I know!"

Emma Gritt, Digital Director at Heart.co.uk

"So grateful to have been introduced to Simone. Her knowledge, expertise and products are second to none. She's not only improved the state of my hair but boosted my confidence and positive outlook. Forever thankful."

BlusherandBabies (Tamara Corin)

"In her book, *Healthy Hair, Happy Body*, Simone gets to the root of 'bad hair days', revealing how our locks act as a mirror, reflecting wellbeing and even happiness. Her story maps her personal journey of discovery of dealing with hair health and loss, and her mission to help others.

Healthy Hair, Happy Body offers diet, health and self-care tips, the benefits of clean living, ideas on prioritising time for a calmer perspective, the power of peaceful 'me time' and unlocking your inner happiness. Simone then shares how to adopt healthy habits to ultimately celebrate a happier version of you...with super healthy hair, of course."

Renate Ruge, travel writer & photographer

Author's Note

From a very young age, I have always had a fear of loss, and a fear of failure. As with most negative elements, my fears are a result of things that have happened in life over the years. My father passed away in 1989, when I was eight years old. He died on impact from severe brain damage and head injuries, as a result of an accident whilst he was in Saudi Arabia. Our life changed overnight, and I can still vividly remember the nightmares that I suffered for years afterwards. So, losing my father definitely had an impact on who and how I am as a person. I am very independent, and don't like to ask for help. This is my way of protecting myself, my way of mentally and physically protecting my future, and my way of protecting my family. I never, ever want to fail, and I am the best person to ensure this.

Following the loss of my father, I watched my mum go from one bad relationship to another. Eventually, she got married to someone whom I hoped would be an amazing father figure, but this turned out not to be the case. Mum was an extremely strong woman, nicknamed "Lady T" or "Ronnie" by most people who knew her. So, when she was later diagnosed with Motor Neurone Disease (MND), and given two years to live, it was quite a shock. She never gave up though, and lived for a full ten more years—eight years longer than the initial diagnosis—passing away when I was twenty-seven.

After that, I had nobody left except my brother and some of my mum's friends. Once again, I felt so lost. More than ever, I needed a parent, especially since I was at a time in life when I was getting settled. For a number of years, I struggled with this, not knowing where to turn, what to do, or how to deal with my grief in a constructive way. But, I have found my way. Everything I have gone through over the course of my lifetime has made me the person I am, and is a constant reminder of why I want to help people and change lives.

My mother and father, and the life they gave me, are the driving force behind my words and my actions. Now, I want to do the same for my two sons, Ashton-Michael and William-Craig. This book is for you, boys. I know you are still young, but one day you will know that you can be whoever you want. Just make sure you are kind, you love with all your heart, and that you have the utmost respect for others—especially women.

Contents

INTRODUCTION

For most of us, the hair-mood phenomenon is all too real. If our hair is brittle, lank, limp, dull, frizzy, wiry or any other adjective that comes to mind when we're having a "bad hair day", we feel terrible. Likewise, when our hair is lustrous, shiny, bouncy, voluminous, cascading, glossy, or velvety, we feel great.

Well, I'll let you in on a secret. Your hair is lank *because* you feel bad. Your hair is glossy *because* you feel good.

You see, it's not your hair that's making you feel good or bad. Of course, receiving comments like, 'Wow, your hair looks amazing' is always nice, but ultimately it's our hair that reflects our mental and physical wellbeing, and *not* the other way round.

So, why is this? Well, the truth is that our hair is not a vital organ. When it comes to our body sharing out its precious nutrients, our hair is at the back of the queue. If we want to guarantee that our hair gets the nutrients it needs, we have to eat well, sleep well, and feel well.

The main aim of this book is to show you that by being healthier and happier, everyone can have great hair. But I also wanted to create a resource for those who are struggling with hair loss, like I did. This was what led me to become an expert in hair loss, nutrition and bioenergetics, and it's the reason I'm perfectly placed to help you in your battle!

Few books exist in the marketplace today that provide a comprehensive understanding of hair health. This black hole in available literature means people who have been affected by poor hair health tend to suffer in silence, or are left to search Google for answers (never the best idea).

To get the most out of this book, I recommend reading it all the way through, from beginning to end, rather than skipping around. Each chapter builds upon the information covered in previous ones. Likewise, each chapter includes a section called "Bringing It All Together", designed to create a big picture in relation to your health, wellbeing, and hair health. Finally, at the end of every chapter, I've included a "Try This" section. This helps you to take the information you've learned, and makes it immediately applicable to your everyday life. There's space to write here, and it can be customised to suit your needs, as you learn more and start figuring out what is best for you.

The bottom line is this, dear reader: if you look after your body, then your body will look after your hair. Throughout this book, I'll show you the best way to do this.

BEFORE WE BEGIN

Let's start with introductions. Hi, my name is Simone Thomas. I've been on an incredible journey. And I feel now is the perfect time to share that journey with you.

At times in my life, I've been in incredible pain, and during others I've shed a lot of tears, but along the way there has also been a lot of love and sunshine.

I'm not a doctor, nor do I profess to be a "wellness warrior". Simply put, my own story has led me to change both my life and my lifestyle. Through it all, I have grown tremendously and learned countless lessons. I've learned that my health, wellbeing and lifestyle are all within my control, and yours is too.

I am about to embark on a potted (I promise!) autobiography, so I suggest you grab a cup of something hot (preferably water with a squeeze of lemon—more on this later!), make yourself comfortable, and I'll begin.

My health issues began at an early age. It started with inflammatory bowel disease (IBD), which caused general discomfort, alongside my first experiences with hair loss. In my late teens and early twenties, I was diagnosed with abnormal cervical cells, which led to a diagnosis of B12-deficiency. It took until my early thirties to discover that I also suffered from endometritis. Any one of these diagnoses alone would cause discomfort and long-term symptoms, but together they caused extreme pain, fatigue, unhealthy weight loss, irregular bleeding, heavy abnormal periods, and pain during intercourse. And, as if all of that wasn't bad enough, another side effect was hair loss. Although I sought medical help, I had to resort to wearing full wigs. As a young woman in her early twenties, and excruciatingly vain, I couldn't decide what was worse, the pain or the hair loss.

I went to get my first hair loss treatment when I was in my late teens, travelling to London to have a semi-permanent wig attached to my existing hair. This was the type of thing that I would keep in day and night, rather than take off for bedtime. To put it bluntly, the experience was awful. I hadn't known at all what to expect, but the process took all day and into the night. And it was a good thing I had a credit card. When it came time to pay, they charged me double what they'd initially quoted me for! I spent the next several years paying off the debt I had incurred. Little did I know, my journey with wigs was only just beginning.

Some might consider it unlucky, but learning of my abnormal cervical cells in my early twenties was a matter of lucky coincidence. In those days, having an annual smear was not commonplace for women. It was generally done only for older women who were already at risk. In fact, despite a large number of younger women being diagnosed with cervical cancer, getting an annual smear didn't become common until the highly publicised death of reality TV star, Jade Goody. In 2009, directly after Goody's death, medical statisticians highlighted a marked increase in the number of women (between the ages of 25-64) getting smears. This figure rose by a huge 12%.

Today, cervical screenings are estimated to save 5,000 lives a year. If every woman attended their screenings regularly, 83% of cervical cancer cases would be prevented. These statistics are both awe-inspiring and shocking, since so many women still don't get a regular smear. Before my incident, I would never have considered getting a smear so young, but thank God I did.

It all started about three months into a new relationship. I didn't feel quite right down below, so I asked my boyfriend how many women he had been with, and if there was anything I should be worried about. At first, he told me that he had only been in a few long-term relationships before me. Yet, when he heard I wasn't feeling well, he got himself checked. The phone call that followed could have come from a sitcom:

'You know how I told you that I had only been in a long-term relationship? Well, that wasn't exactly true. After I broke up with my previous long-term girlfriend, I had a few one-night stands...but they were all very posh, so I'm sure there's nothing to worry about.'

Turned out, it was something to worry about! I went to the nurse at the doctor's surgery, and she tested me for STDs. In the process, she did a smear, just to be thorough. I came back with chlamydia, which is common and easily treatable. Of course, I immediately called up my boyfriend and gave him the boot! But, what concerned the doctors more, was my abnormally high cervical cell count.

At the time, I was preparing for an upcoming holiday to Egypt, but they told me I had to go straight to hospital to perform more tests and receive treatment. This was also when they discovered my B-12 deficiency. Operations, including surgery to remove the pre-cancer cervical cells, did nothing to relieve my symptoms. However, it was the encouragement I needed to try and treat myself.

Following numerous nutritionists' advice, I followed an anti-inflammatory diet. We will talk more about this later, but in essence, it's a diet that cuts out food known to aggravate already existing inflammation. This diet helped my symptoms dramatically, although it didn't cure the underlying cause.

About a week after breaking up with my boyfriend, I called him and said that it might not have been such a bad thing that he'd (inadvertently) given me an STD. We got back together, and even went so far as to get engaged. In the end, it didn't work out, although we were on-off again a few times before finally calling it quits. He remains a good friend to this day. Without him, I wouldn't be here, because I would never have received my diagnosis or removed those pre-cancer cells. But, if we had got married, my initials would have been STD—which really would have been the icing on the cake!

Ten years before sitting down to write this book, following the death of my mother, I decided to rent a small apartment, choosing to be near my brother and his family in Dorset. It was then that I noticed more extreme hair loss, and thus I reverted to wearing full wigs. From the time I was diagnosed, to the passing of my mother, my symptoms (including hair loss) fluctuated, so I went through various stages of wigs. I tried extensions, volumisers (half-wigs that clipped in), integrated systems that attached semi-permanently, and day-to-day wigs that I could take on and off like a pair of shoes. My age and lack of money meant that the quality of my wigs and extensions weren't always what they should have been. The same applied to my diet. I often ate McDonald's and drank with my friends, none of which helped my conditions.

Despite my inconsistent focus on nutrition and diet, my hair loss condition really troubled me. Sadly, neither diagnosis, sympathy, nor solutions were forthcoming. Searching for answers, I began to realise that there was in fact a serious gap in the market for a specialist hair salon, where men, women and children with hair loss issues could be supported. So, I went out and researched, studied, and learned everything there was to know about hair loss systems. As a result, my company "Makeup, Wigs & Hair" (M.W.A.H.) was born in 2012.

Within months, M.W.A.H. was welcoming women, men, transgenders, and children who came to the salon to enjoy professional makeup application, beauty services, nail care, big bouncy blow-dries, and the opportunity to delve into our huge stock of hair extensions, hair systems, and wigs.

From day one, I felt I had really found my niche. I loved it! Seeing our clients smile with newfound confidence when their new wig or hair system was fitted, was a dream come true. I was finally making a difference in people's lives, in a way that I wished someone could have done when I was at the height of my hair loss. As time went on, clients began to rely not only on my services, but on myself and the support system that I had created. I realised that, like me, they needed more than cosmetic help. So, I extended my studies and took a course to study nutrition and bioenergetics. M.W.A.H. was such a success, that within three years I relocated to a two-storey building, which became the "Simone Thomas" flagship, soon employing a team of 22 people.

At Simone Thomas, on a daily basis, we offer our clients a 90-minute consultation which analyses their medical history, diet, and lifestyle. Afterwards, we examine the scalp and hair under a microscope. Through our research, we've discovered that there are an enormous range of factors which can contribute to hair loss and scalp health, including poor diet, drug use, autoimmune disorders, hormone imbalances, and many other lifestyle choices that you wouldn't necessarily associate with hair.

My own studies in nutrition and weight loss management have only confirmed my theory that almost all of my clients' ailments lead right back to their gut. And it makes sense too. All diseases originate in the gut, so why aren't we paying it more attention? The old adage, "You are what you eat" could not be truer! Fatigue, skin complaints, and poor sleep patterns are all signs of inflammation caused by the food we eat. Put simply—eat well and your body will perform well. Over the years, I have witnessed so many dramatic changes in our clients' hair loss conditions and general wellbeing, just by them addressing their diets and lifestyles. I also believe that I've found a cure to ease my own condition.

I relentlessly continue my studies throughout the UK, Europe, and the USA in order to learn as much about the gut, nutrition and hair loss as possible. It's a fact that a healthy gut doesn't just empower general health—it can manage more serious ailments too.

Having shared and practised with such successful results, I have been urged to share my findings with a wider audience. So here it is: *Healthy Hair, Happy Body*—a book that is literally my personal edit of the best advice I've ever used and given. Hopefully, you'll reap the benefits too.

Happy Reading xx

Chapter One: My Process

If you are anything like me—you are tired! I'm totally aware that I am not the only person who is multi-tasking! This is especially the case since I'm a mum to two young boys. In 2017, the father of my boys nearly died from a brain seizure. On top of this, he's surfing mad, and used to go for a walk on the wild side; so I know first-hand how exhausting everyday life can be. In addition, I'm MD of hair loss clinics and hairdressing salons, with my own range of award-winning wellness products, and—oh yes, author of this book. So yes, sometimes I feel frazzled!

In today's culture, most people are familiar with feeling either too busy, too overwhelmed, or simply too tired. In fact, studies have reported that one in three Britons reports suffering from insomnia. We live in a fast-paced world, where we must often make sacrifices of one kind or another. Too often, especially for working parents, this means sacrificing our own wellbeing.

Luckily, I live by the coast—and the only way I can survive my week is by rising every other day at 5:30 a.m. This ensures that I get very valued "me" time for at least forty-five minutes before my darling boys wake up. In that time, I ensure that I am "still" and choose to do exactly what I want to do. If I can pull myself away from my really bad online shopping habit, I read quietly, meditate, or sometimes simply leave the house and go for a walk along the beach, do a spot of exercise, or just "be". You can gain far more from getting up a bit earlier than having a lie-in. Believe me—I can't express how good it feels to have that time to myself (and the shopping bags to open!).

Healthy Hair, Happy Body

I first came to discover the power of "quiet time" by accident. After the birth of my first son, I struggled. With my mother and father having passed away when I was younger, I didn't have a great support system in place. Just three days after my son was born, I had to jump right back into work. I'd won a prestigious award as the "Entrepreneur of Great Britain"—which would mean amazing press coverage—so I couldn't turn down this opportunity, especially as a relatively new business. Of course, I didn't leave my son entirely, but bringing him into meetings and finding breaks to feed him didn't exactly make anything easier! Having a child is a huge adjustment, even for mothers who are lucky enough to have some time at home, but caring for a newborn baby whilst building a business proved quite overwhelming, to say the least.

I can remember driving home, about three months into motherhood, thinking that I could just plough into oncoming traffic. My mantra was, 'No one loves me. No one cares. The world would be a better place without me.' The words seemed to play on repeat. Anyone familiar with this is probably shouting, 'It's postpartum depression!' However, I wasn't at all aware of this condition, so I didn't know what was wrong with me. All I knew was that these thoughts and feelings were unlike anything I had previously experienced.

When I finally called my doctor, he didn't even ask me to come into the surgery. He diagnosed me over the phone with postpartum depression, and immediately called in a prescription for anti-depressants. After I picked the pills up, I studied them in my hand, debating if I should take my first dose. Before I did, I spoke to my brother. I broke down, telling him everything I had been thinking and feeling for weeks on end. In response, my brother urged me not to take the anti-depressants. He worried that while they might help the symptoms, they wouldn't help the underlying issues I was facing, and then it would be too late to stop taking them. So, instead of using the pills, I took a holiday. I planned a two-week getaway to Greece at a luxury spa, as a way for me to reset. Whilst at the airport, I walked through WHSmith. My eye was drawn to a book called *The Miracle Morning: The Not So Obvious Secret Guaranteed To Transform Your* Life, by Hal Elrod. I spent my holiday reading it, and it did, in fact, change my life! I came back from my trip a different person, committed to enacting the advice in the book.

Elrod's book isn't for everyone, but the big takeaway message is that by giving yourself an hour every morning, whether you spend that time meditating, doing yoga, reading a book, or just enjoying your coffee with the sunrise, you will not only be a happier person but a more productive person as well. A lot of people will say some variation of, 'Bloody hell, I don't even have two minutes to pee in peace!' I get that, I truly do, but it was this mentality of putting everyone else first, pushing myself to the limits, and never slowing down, that pushed *me* to the brink of depression and suicidal thoughts.

Healthy Hair, Happy Body

You have to make the choice. It's about restructuring your life to reshuffle your priorities. Take a long, hard look at your day. How can you re-define your time or the activities you choose, in order to fit in some time for yourself? We are all the same on this planet. We have twenty-four hours each day to make our choices. The question is, how do you want to be accountable in those twenty-four hours?

In the past, I didn't always give myself permission to find the time for me, and that is exactly what taking care of yourself requires: permission. Take heed of your frazzled-ness and use it as your prompt to recharge. Nothing is better than being awake and aware of the fact that you are recharging! Now, I manage to find time for myself at least two mornings a week. On those days, I feel like a different person. I am better able to make good choices throughout the day, and I face my day with a calmer perspective.

Once you start trying this simple exercise i.e. finding time for yourself, you will be able to power through your day. Not only will you be happier in the long term, but I can guarantee that you will feel healthier. If a little guilt does creep in, always remind yourself that in order to take care of others, you need to take care of yourself first.

When I started nourishing myself and showing myself even the teeniest moments of love, like buying a new lipstick or sipping my morning hot water and lemon without children at my feet, I immediately felt such a sense of wellbeing. It was as though I was tapping into an energy within me that had laid dormant for far too long. These wonderful endorphins are in all of us. Even when we feel absolutely depleted, a simple act such as a blow-dry, manicure, going to the gym, or lifting weights can re-energise you. If, like me, you have an endless to-do list and demands from countless people, then you have no option but to stay living in the fast lane. But whilst in the fast lane, I urge you to pull over and take stock of what is really important to you. Then, it's up to you to decide what to do with your energy and how you want to run your life.

Go on, try it.

> If we didn't take care of ourselves, we wouldn't be in a position to take care of others. So, there's nothing selfish about looking after you.

Of course, these are just temporary "fixes". When I embarked on my journey of transformative self-care, it took me to a completely different level. The greatest thing I learned was how to nourish myself from within, and not just on the surface. Learning *how* to take time for yourself, is an important first step. You must acknowledge the value of your own wellbeing as an equal priority to all of your other responsibilities. Then, you have to give yourself permission—permission to fit *yourself* into your own life. Everything that follows in this book stems from the idea that your health—both physically and mentally—is worth it, and that you have the power right now to change this for the better. It won't happen overnight, but when you come to this realisation, you'll immediately love this new way of living.

Remember—you've got to love yourself to do it. xxx

> The longest relationship you have in your life is with yourself.

Bringing It All Together

From the outset, making time each day to take care of yourself can seem like an impossible task. But, in the end, the journey you are beginning today will be worth it in the long run. As I mentioned earlier, your hair is often the first indicator of your overall health, and this is especially true when it comes to your stress levels. If you are allowing your day to be consumed by the needs of others, whilst ignoring your own, the chances are your stress levels are only getting worse. Too often, we ignore our stress as just an inevitable part of life that we can't do anything about.

It's important to start rewriting these ideas, or you will start seeing and feeling the side effects of your stress. Stress hormones are powerful chemicals, originally intended to jump-start your body when in danger, enabling you to fight, or run away and stay safe. In modern times, those same stress hormones are wreaking havoc on our systems. When we live in a constant state of stress, our bodies are always on high alert, and our hormones are always in flux. This creates an environment that is not conducive to hair growth. In order to set the stage for optimal hair growth, as well as healthy skin and nails, you have to start prioritising your own needs and getting your stress under control.

Try This

This chapter is all about recognising your own needs for self-care. The first step toward self-care is recognising *why* you need it. Not why I need it, or why your friends think you should be getting it, but why *you* need it. Take some time to think about why you picked up this book. Was it simply to improve your hair and skin? Was it because you felt out of control and wanted to make a change?

Start your first "Try This" by writing down your goals and intentions with this book. If you can only think of one thing that you want to accomplish by the end of this book, that's okay, but keep this section in mind as you learn more. Come back whenever you think of a new goal, and write it here until you have at least five goals.

1. _____

2. _____

3. _____

4. _____

5. _____

Now, back to our self-care! I don't want you to simply nod your head agreeably whilst reading, only to move on without implementing anything we have talked about. Self-care takes a conscious effort. It isn't going to magically fall into your lap or be gifted to you by someone else.

I want you to choose **TWO** days this week where you can set your alarm for fifteen minutes earlier. I know, it sounds hard. But, if you didn't get enough sleep to begin with, then that fifteen minutes is not going to make or break how tired you feel.

Next, I want you to plan exactly how you're going to spend those first fifteen minutes of your day, and it *isn't* going to be pulling up your phone to check work emails or social media. It *is* going to be healthy tasks, setting you up for a positive, calmer day. If you can't think of anything, you can borrow directly from my routine:

First, I take some calming, deep breaths to relax myself, pushing my day's "to-do" list out of my head. Then, I get in the shower, which always ends with a burst of freezing cold. I am sure you are saying to yourself, 'But Simone, a freezing shower doesn't sound relaxing.' I urge you to try it. The cold water increases your heart rate and gives you an instant burst of energy to start your day. Cold showers have also been proven to improve weight loss, skin and hair, immunity, mood, and sooth muscles. So, give it a try!

After my shower, I always make my bed. This sets me up for the rest of the day (maybe that is my education from Private Royal Naval School coming out!). I finish it all off with a cup of hot water with lemon, and drink my hot water while sitting. I make sure not to multitask during my time to myself, otherwise it defeats the purpose.

Here are some more ideas to try:

- Read a book.

- Go for a brisk walk.

- Meditate (see chapter seven for tips on how to get started with meditation practice).

- Do a ten-minute yoga routine.

- Set an intention for the day. An intention can be as simple as saying, 'I will be grateful today.' Or, it can be more specific to your life situation. Essentially, an intention is a short, one-line sentence that outlines your purpose and focus for the day, and which you can easily go back to later, in order to reset yourself and refocus on your personal goals.

- Write in a journal.

Chapter Two: FOR GUT'S SAKE

Your gut is the "mothership" of your whole body. I know what you're probably thinking: isn't my brain the "mothership"? After all, your brain is what allows you to think, and is the hub that connects various systems together. Although that may be true, the overall wellbeing and harmony of your systems is determined by your gut. It is your gut that is responsible for the healthy functioning of every part of your body (including, as a matter of fact, your brain). From hair loss and brittle nails to bloating and skin problems, it all begins in the gut. It used to be that everyone blamed long-term health problems on your genes, but now more and more research is being dedicated to the substantial link between your gut and your health.

I cannot overstate how vital the connection between body and gut is to your health. It is the job of your gut to effectively absorb nutrients from the food you eat, remove toxins, and regulate your immune system, but in doing those things it ends up achieving so much more. It is in our intestines that bacteria flourish. There are between 75 to 125 trillion bacteria living in your gut right now. I know, gross, but we actually have a unique, symbiotic relationship with these bacteria, that can create all kinds of healthy or unhealthy side effects. Research overwhelmingly shows that the more healthy bacteria you have, the better off you are. This is mostly because each bacterium has its own job to do, from breaking down food to boosting immunity, and other such tasks. The higher the healthy bacteria count in your gut, the more efficiently your gut can do all of its many jobs.

A Gut Imbalance

So, this all sounds wonderful so far. We have these happy little bacteria living inside of us, working away to create a healthy eco-system inside our bodies. Yet, if out of balance, this "mothership" of ours can really wreak havoc on our system. Meaning, if you have too few types of bacteria or too many of one type and not enough of another, there's trouble ahead, and this trouble will manifest in problems with your body. For example, if your hair is falling out in clumps when you wash it in the shower, it may be because your gut isn't balanced. Have you ever taken a dose of antibiotics, only to end up with diarrhoea or a yeast infection? That is because the antibiotics kill bacteria. That includes the bacteria in your stomach, leaving your whole system out of whack. And, it's not just our hair and scalp that's affected. Fatigue, skin complaints, and poor sleep patterns are all signs of inflammation in the gut too.

So often, we go through life with ailments that we just assume are normal parts of modern living. The prime example, of course, being a feeling of ever-present exhaustion, but this can also include upset stomachs or bloating after a meal. Few people make the connection between what they are eating and how they are feeling. But in fact, the food we eat and how our individual bodies react to it, is often both the cause and the cure. Eat well and you'll perform well!

Mind and Gut Connection

We have been talking a lot about the physical side effects of your balanced (or imbalanced) gut, but there is a clear link between your gut health and your mental wellbeing too.

For the majority of us, it isn't hard to recognise the power of the gut, even on a daily basis. Most people will be familiar with the phrase "gut feeling", which is where your gut tells you what the right decision is. Or, perhaps you are going into a big, important presentation and your stomach starts doing flips. Those feelings *are* the power of the gut. You get those queasy stomach feelings because your gut carries responses directly to and from the brain. This is why it is often referred to as the "second brain". The gut houses the enteric nervous system (ENS) which contains more nerve cells than even your spinal cord. The purpose of this nervous system is to allow us to feel what is happening inside the gut. Your "second brain" may not contribute to your thought process in the traditional sense, but it certainly does communicate in a big way. Those "gut feelings" are our guts reacting to stress in a real and physical way. When people say things like "trust your gut" they aren't wrong. Your gut really is trying to tell you things! With such a large nervous system living there, it's not surprising then that when we're stressed and run-down, we get an upset stomach.

Modern-day stress is an interesting beast, and is far more complicated than our bodies were designed to handle effectively. Most of us have heard of the "flight or fight" response. When we face a stressful or scary situation, like narrowly missing a car accident or presenting in front of a large crowd, our body releases adrenalin. This is important when you have to react fast to avoid that accident or be laser-focused in your meeting. The only problem is when our stress lasts longer than it should. All too often, we are in a perpetual state of high stress. We aren't allowing our minds or bodies the time they need to normalise.

So, now you know that your gut *can* react to your mood, but did you know that your gut can *affect* your mood too? Your gut contains 95% of your serotonin. For those of you not in the "know", serotonin is your natural "happy" neurotransmitter. That means that if your gut is unhealthy, out of balance, or inflamed, then it can't produce serotonin. As a result, your mood will plummet. Serotonin has also been linked to regulating your sleep cycles. Whilst on the subject of mood—the truth is that sometimes what we mistake as depression is simply a signal from our body that we aren't taking care of it properly. That isn't to say that symptoms of depression shouldn't be taken seriously, but as I learned from personal experience, there may be underlying problems that won't be cured by a pill.

In addition to supporting our immune system and producing serotonin, the gut produces more than two dozen hormones that influence our body, impacting everything from our appetite to our mood. Hormones can be really complex. Often, when doctors and nutritionists talk about them, hormones sound like mystic forces that we can't possibly understand. In truth, at their most basic, hormones are the messengers of the body; controlling and managing sexual health, organ function, energy levels, and growth, among many other things. When hormones are out of balance, we can often tell right away that something doesn't "feel" quite right, but it is harder to pinpoint exactly where that feeling originates. We may assume we aren't getting enough sleep, that we are getting a cold, or that we are simply stressed. Often, however, the culprit is a hormone imbalance Since many hormones are produced directly in the gut, when the gut is out of balance, these hormones are out of balance too. Suffice to say, we need our serotonin, hormones, and all the things a healthy gut provides for us! So, come on now—let's start looking after it!

What Is the Gut?

After all this explanation of why the gut is so incredibly important, you might still be wondering, 'What the heck is the gut though?' Well, when I talk about the gut, I am referring to your whole digestive system, including your stomach, small intestine, large intestine, liver, and gallbladder. Your gut is the system that is responsible for taking in and breaking down food into useful nutrients and waste. Your gut's job begins as soon as food or drink enters through your mouth. Just about everything your body needs, is processed by the gut. This also means, however, that anything you put into your body plays a role in how your body functions, and therefore affects how you feel.

How Can We Improve Our Gut?

The answer to this question is simple. Eat better foods! If you are not feeding your gut with the right types and varieties of food, it can't possibly fuel your body and mind. It's a bit like putting petrol in a diesel car. Studies have found that unhealthy diets lead to 89,900 deaths a year in the UK. That equals out to about one in six deaths, all attributed to not eating the right kinds of foods. Eating healthier can, quite literally, save your life.

Of course, for anyone who is new to thinking about their health or their diet, this advice may be a case of easier said than done. Fixing your gut and eating healthier generally requires a change in diet. When I use the word diet in this book, I use it in the traditional sense, referring simply to the types of food you eat, rather than the newer understanding of the word, which means restricting calories or following a special plan. Changing your diet starts with eliminating foods which promote the growth of harmful bacteria. The next step is adding in the foods that your diet may be lacking, such as whole grains, fruits, vegetables, and high-quality protein. The study mentioned earlier found that the deadliest diet woes were a low intake of whole grains, fruits, nuts, and vegetables, and a high intake of salt. (If that sounds like the description of a "happy meal" to you, then you are correct. It's the fast-food epidemic.)

The next logical question, of course, is 'what is a healthy diet?' Ever since people started thinking about their food, and even more so with the advent of social media, there seems to be one fad diet after another. A lot of this is geared directly towards weight loss. But, it is important to remember that weight loss plans don't equate to a healthy gut. While getting to or maintaining a healthy weight is always an important step towards health, it is important to remember that weight loss alone may not resolve hair, skin, sleep, or mood issues. Eating 1,200 calories a day to lose weight means nothing for your gut health, if those 1,200 calories are crisps and ice cream.

In truth, a healthy diet is far simpler than every fad will have you believe. It consists of plenty of fresh vegetables, fruits, quality protein, and the assistance of probiotics (more on supplements later). Remember that the main function of our digestive systems is to transport vital nutrients into our internal organs and other systems. For our bodies to function, they need a complete range of nutrients contained in the food and drink we consume. These are fats, proteins, carbohydrates, fibre, water, minerals, and vitamins. As our hair is not a vital organ or tissue, it simply does not receive top priority when it comes to being on the receiving end of nutrients, so it often needs extra help, especially if you aren't even getting enough nutrients to sustain all of your vital functions.

Nutrients You Need

In the next chapters, we will discuss how to make healthy eating into a daily, achievable, lifestyle goal. But for now, let's take a quick look at the basic nutrients to start creating a positive impact on gut health (and therefore hair health). Low levels of the following nutrients could have an impact on your health and your hair, and stop you from being the best version of you. You can fast track your wellbeing, by introducing a diet high in:

Nutrient	What It's For	What It's Found In
A	Healthy vision. Improves bone, skin, and immune function.	Sweet potatoes, milk, cheese, liver, spinach, carrots, eggs.
B1	Supports nervous system, brain function, muscles, heart, stomach, intestines, and the flow of electrolytes.	Cauliflower, liver, oranges, eggs, potatoes, asparagus, kale.
B3	Increases good cholesterol (HDL) and lowers bad cholesterol. Helps convert food to energy. Keeps skin, hair, and nervous system healthy.	Liver, chicken, turkey, salmon, brown rice, enriched breakfast cereal, peanuts.

B6	Promotes healthy metabolism, liver, nerve system, mood, and brain function. Promotes healthy skin and eye health.	Beef, turkey, tuna, pistachios, pinto beans, avocado, molasses, sunflower seeds, sesame seeds.
B12	Helps make DNA. Prevents anaemia and encourages healthy blood cells.	Beef, clams, fish, meat, poultry, eggs, breakfast cereals.
C	Growth and repair of skin tissues. Repairs cartilage, bones and teeth, aids in iron absorption, and acts as an antioxidant—boosting your immune system.	Kale, bell peppers, thyme, parsley, kiwi, broccoli, oranges.
D	Promotes bone growth, prevents breast cancer, colon cancer, prostate cancer, heart disease, depression, and weight gain.	Salmon, sardines, tuna, oysters, shrimp, eggs, mushrooms.
E	Antioxidant, helping with healthy skin, nails, hair, and eyes. Prevents cancer, heart disease, diabetes, Alzheimer's, and cataracts.	Sunflower seeds, almonds, avocado, spinach, butternut squash, kiwi, broccoli.

Arginine	Amino acid that promotes healthy liver, skin, joints, and muscles. Improves the immune system and regulates hormones and blood sugar.	Turkey, pork, chicken, pumpkin seeds, chickpeas, peanuts.
Manganese	Healthy bones, disease prevention, hormone regulation, improved metabolism.	Nuts, legumes, seeds, tea, whole grains, and green leafy vegetables.
Magnesium	Prevents depression, high blood pressure, and heart disease. Improves brain function, nerve cells and memory.	Seeds, cashews, dark leafy greens, salmon, tuna, escargot.
Selenium	Protects against damage, acts as antioxidant, regulates blood pressure. Supports immune system, anti-aging, and thyroid.	Brazil nuts, fish, ham, enriched pasta, whole wheat, eggs.
Zinc	Improves immune system, makes proteins and DNA, and supports healing.	Oysters, wild rice, shiitake, pumpkin seeds, whole wheat, oatmeal, lentils, beef.

I am proof that with the right diet and the correct lifestyle changes, practically anyone can get back into peak condition. I have experienced first-hand the power of nutrition in tackling various ailments. By feeding my family with the correct probiotics and food types/groups, I have been able to find a solution for us all.

Supplements

All of the nutrients I mentioned can be found in the foods you eat. But, if you looked at the above table and felt overwhelmed, then that's totally okay. It would be virtually impossible to develop a daily meal plan that included at least one item, in enough quantities, to meet the recommended intake for each nutrient I described. That's where supplements come in. Our busy lifestyles don't always allow us to eat as healthily as we'd like, which is why I created my range of wellbeing supplements, including my SkinQuencher for collagen, Ginkgo Biloba B+, and Biotin Brilliance. They incorporate a high-strength probiotic, plus an all-in-one alkalising super green, daily nourishment supplement, which work together to maintain a healthy gut function.

If you're still not sure, think of supplements as a kind of cheat sheet. They allow you to focus your efforts, helping you to get healthy, while still making sure you're getting all the essential nutrients you need. In other words, you won't be spending all your time calculating the micro-nutrients of everything you eat, because you will *already* be getting them through supplements. Don't forget to include a probiotic supplement in your daily regime too, in order to replenish your levels of gut bacteria. My award-winning "Everyday Wellbeing Supplements" can help with this.

To streamline finding the right vitamins for my clients, I've created a line of supplements that can be found at www.simonethomaswellness.com. All of them are aligned with the health and nutrition goals of this book.

Summing It All Up

Every person's healing journey will be unique. There are formulas you can follow at the onset, but each person's needs, body, and gut are different. For example, if I have dairy, I know that I will almost instantly feel bloated with a loud gurgling stomach. Meanwhile, other people drink half a gallon of milk per day and feel fine. The key is to think of this book and the advice it contains as a road map, to get you started on the path to health. When you first start out, you will probably follow the "Try This" sections precisely, without any personal modifications. But, as you learn more about your body and your preferences, you will start making this journey your own.

As you do start finding your way, keep in mind the key ingredients to health. Often, the things that ail us are merely symptoms of larger, underlying problems within our gut. Therefore, be mindful of the advice you get and the pills you are suggested to take. It may be that you are treating symptoms rather than the cause. Pills might make you feel better in the short term, but underneath that, you'll still be suffering. You wouldn't construct a building by starting on the top floor, and you shouldn't try to construct long-lasting health that way either.

Bringing It All Together

If you follow the advice laid out in this book, you will start getting healthy and feeling better, but it will also help you *look* better! A balanced gut means a balanced body, and that includes your hair, nails, and skin. As the link between your gut health and your overall health becomes more and more apparent, so too does the link between your gut health and your hair. It may seem a little crazy to imagine that what goes on in your intestines affects what happens on the top of your head, but that is exactly the case!

Hair growth relies primarily on three things: blood flow, nutrients, and hormones. Your gut is responsible for maintaining and promoting healthy blood flow, supplying essential nutrients, and regulating your hormones. What's even more interesting is the link between probiotics and healthy hair. Probiotics are living microorganisms that replenish and balance the microbiome already living there, keeping everything healthy. Using mice, scientists discovered that probiotic supplements can increase hair growth by 106%, with enormous differentiations in hair growth between the mice who were given the supplements, compared to mice who weren't.

This study tells us how incredibly important the health of our gut is in growing hair, and how important taking a probiotic supplement can be to the health of our gut!

Try This

Before you can change your diet, you must make a concentrated effort to understand it. Spend the next three days writing down everything that you put into your diet. This isn't about calories, so you don't have to cheat. Use the chart below to keep a log of your diet over three days. Be honest with yourself as you keep your log. The purpose of this is to learn, grow, and reflect.

Day 1 Date:			
Food or drink	Approx amount	Time of day	How you feel

Day 2	Date:		
Food or drink	Approx amount	Time of day	How you feel

Day 3	Date:		
Food or drink	Approx amount	Time of day	How you feel

Healthy Hair, Happy Body

When your three days is up, I want you to take a look at the foods you ate. For the sake of making this easier, put each food and drink into one of two categories: "Good" or "Bad". Good foods mean whole, natural, fruits, vegetables, proteins, nuts, legumes. Bad means processed, sugary, fast foods.

Once you have done that, look through your list and compare it to my chart from the "Nutrients You Need". How often do you think you are hitting your nutrient count? What are some of your weaknesses when it comes to food? What kind of "bad" or unhealthy foods do you indulge in? Is there any obvious connection between the food you ate and how you felt, whether it be physical i.e. bloated, or emotional i.e. anxious?

Over the course of this book, we are going to talk a lot about how your body works and what kinds of fuel your body needs. Keep this food diary handy, because we will use it again to start making adjustments to your life and diet, that you can put into practise straight away. Remember, this book is about changing the way you think about yourself. Together, we will help you to make better lifestyle choices, improving the way you feel and allowing your hair to flourish!

Chapter Three: CLEAN LIVING

Now that I've explained the importance of a healthy gut, it's time to make that goal a reality. As I mentioned in the last chapter, when we break down what the gut needs most, it comes down to "clean living". I am sure you have heard the words "eating clean" and "clean living" before, to the point where they've almost become a cliché. But, what do these terms really mean? Why does clean living matter? And what about all those celebrities talking about carbs, or the Ketogenic diet vs Paleo diet, juice-cleansing, and macros? Let's slow it down and take a step back!

The truth is, there are as many different diets as there are people on earth. Before you can start adjusting how *you* eat, you must first understand the basic foundations of what is healthy. It wasn't until I had children of my own that I began to understand the importance of clean living. At six weeks old, my son nearly died from the rotavirus, which caused his organs to shut down. I knew I had to pull out all the stops to save him. Sadly, the virus and subsequent trauma caused damage to both his digestive tract and vagus nerve, which runs the length of the back and interfaces with the parasympathetic system, controlling the heart, lungs, and digestive tract. This meant that even after the initial danger had passed, he still struggled with inflammation, pain, digestion issues, and many other health-related problems.

In the same way that I did when my own inflammation endometritis reared its head, I took a hard look at my son's diet. Small changes over time made a huge difference to his health, how he felt, and his mood. Now, with the right diet and medical care, he can lead a happy life.

Why Clean Living?

Just as we shouldn't underestimate the power of the gut on our overall health, neither should we underestimate the idea of clean living. What we put into our bodies can and does have a huge impact on our health. Most negative food-related side effects come from the underlying issue of an unhealthy gut. But, there is more to it than that. How can you expect to feel energised, healthy, and positive if you are essentially starving your body of the real nutrition it needs? Your body needs fuel to maintain basic functions, let alone perform at a high level. That fuel comes in the form of the food you eat.

When you start thinking about the food you eat as fuel—something that can either help you perform better or leave you run down—or in the worst case create side effects (yep, some foods can cause negative side effects just like you read on the side of a drug label!), it is easier to start understanding why clean living is important.

The benefits of clean eating are so plentiful that a quick Google search will result in at least ten examples before you have even clicked on a link. I am going to come back to this idea time and again, but essentially when you eat clean, your body has the fuel it needs to both thrive and fight.

You've got to nourish to flourish.

What Is Clean Living?

"Clean foods" are those that haven't been drastically changed from their natural form. For example, an apple in a bowl still resembles the apple on the tree, whereas a crisp looks nothing like a potato, as it has been heavily processed. Clean living means not eating anything with added artificial flavour, and not eating foods that last for months and months. If the food expires naturally in the fridge or the cupboard, then that's a sign it's safe to eat!

When I'm shopping, I always look at the label. If I can count more than seven ingredients, it doesn't hit my trolley. This extends to products containing ingredients that I can neither pronounce nor recognise. It also really helps to focus on products where sugar isn't the main ingredient, or in the first three listed.

In line with the above, a clean kitchen is the heart and soul of your clean lifestyle. It is the space in your home where you keep the ingredients and tools you will need to make clean meals, helping to nourish you and your family. Keeping your kitchen well stocked is one of the most important ways to make clean eating easy and fun. Having a wide variety of ingredients and condiments around will also take the stress out of preparing recipes.

While you may be making a mental list of all the junk food that you can no longer eat, take heart. Clean living is actually the easiest type of "diet" or nutritional change you can make. There aren't restrictions on how much you can eat, and it doesn't require you to starve yourself or give up an entire category of food. Instead, it is all about getting to the source of the nutrition you need. You are no longer eating piles of food while starving yourself nutritionally. The rules are simple, easy to follow and easy to start fitting into your life right away.

Clean Eating Rules:

1. **Fresh.** No preservatives that keep food viable after an apocalypse.

2. **Whole.** Food should be recognisable and as close to its natural form as possible.

3. **Real.** No artificial boosters and "natural" ingredients that change the colour, flavour, or consistency of your food.

4. **Delicious.** Explore new varieties of fruits, vegetables, cooking styles, and spices to make delicious and nutritious meals.

My Guide to Clean Living

The idea of clean eating and living can seem overwhelming, especially if you have sustained yourself on fast food up until this point. But, fear not. I am here to help you incorporate it into your life. You will find that if you commit, you will adapt quickly—and goodness me you'll start to feel so much better! Clean living will become pretty intuitive when you follow my little rule book.

1. **Eat First Thing.** Start your day by ensuring that you eat within the first hour of waking, otherwise your body will go into "stress" mode.

2. **Wait on the Caffeine.** Don't have your first caffeinated drink (tea or coffee) until 11:00 a.m. Instead, opt for a cup of hot water with a squeeze of lemon. Your circadian rhythm (the natural process that regulates your sleep and wake cycle) all but guarantees that when you first wake up, you will have the most energy. As the day goes on, however, the hormones released when you first woke (that help you feel refreshed and energetic) will start to wane. This means that you don't actually need a cup of coffee in the morning, and in fact you may be throwing off your rhythms if you do. So, wait until the mid-morning lull (if it ever comes!).

3. **Take Your Time.** Take time when you eat, and always put your phone away. Sit down and eat leisurely—you'll get an immense feeling of satisfaction and fullness. This also prevents over-eating. It takes

fifteen to twenty minutes for your brain to receive the signal from your stomach that it has received enough food. If you are eating too quickly, by the time your brain gets word that you've had enough, you have already overindulged. This is coupled with the added risk of acid reflux and indigestion. So, slow it down!

4. **Prep Work is Key.** Take time to prep your food. Ideally, you want to start from scratch with each meal. Steam or bake your food as opposed to microwaving. Microwaved food is as good as useless if you are looking for any health-boosting antioxidants. In short, antioxidants help prevent cell damage and can even help repair cells. When we microwave our fresh produce and vegetables, the fast-acting waves that help make our food hot also kill off those antioxidants. It takes less than fifteen minutes to steam a head of broccoli. So, with a little pre-planning, you will have a fresh meal in thirty minutes. For anyone struggling with what to eat or how to cook, check out NutriHome https://simonethomaswellness.com/blogs/nutrihome which is filled with recipes and advice.

5. **The Miracle of Water**. Drink a glass of water at least thirty minutes before eating a meal. This will help you avoid overeating and keep your digestive system healthy, maximising the uptake of beneficial beauty nutrients.

6. **About Snacks**. If you start craving a snack, try drinking a glass of water instead. Don't quench your thirst on fizzy caffeinated drinks

and alcohol, as these cause spikes in blood sugar levels, which can make you feel hungrier than you are. Always check your hunger pangs by drinking a glass of water, as the hormones that trigger food cravings and thirst are the same! So, maybe you were just thirsty after all? This doesn't mean you should starve yourself though. Instead, determine if you are really hungry or not. So many of us have forgotten what real hunger feels like, because we've spent so long eating out of boredom or because it was simply time. Check in with your body. Make sure you understand what it is telling you.

7. **When to Eat.** Maintain your blood sugar levels throughout the day by eating approximately every two to three hours. Both snacks and main meals should include protein and carbohydrates (natural carbohydrates like veggies and fruit, not a piece of white bread). This combination slows the release of sugar from carbohydrates into your bloodstream, preventing hunger pangs and providing a steady supply of energy for your body. If you choose to snack on fruit, don't reach for the juiciest piece—that's the one bursting with sugar!

8. **When to Eat, Part 2.** Always eat between a twelve-hour window, 7:00 a.m-7:00 p.m. This gives your digestive system, your gut, and your body time to rest and process all the nutrients you fed them throughout the day.

9. **Food Diversity**. All vegetables were created equal but different. They all have different combinations of nutrients. This means that in order to get the most well-balanced diet, you should be eating a wide variety of different vegetables. To do this, always have some herbs growing, and add them to your salads. Have a vegetable box delivered. This will ensure that you not only introduce new vegetables to your diet, but also that these vegetables are locally sourced and in season. Consume the entire asparagus, not just the tip. Likewise, consume the trunk of the broccoli, not just the crown.

10. **Organic**. Where possible, always eat organic. Non-organic produce is likely to have been sprayed with pesticides, leaving toxic by-products that often can't be removed by washing, scrubbing, or peeling. On a related note, I have a fantastic podcast episode on this very subject, which was done alongside the brilliant Barbara Cox. You can check this out by searching for "Living Life Well with Simone Thomas". https://simonethomaswellness.com/blogs/podcast

11. **Invest in a Juicer.** Juicing is a great way to get the nutrients from lots of fruits and vegetables, all in one little glass. If you find you aren't eating enough vegetables, simply turn them into juice instead!

Seasonal Fruits and Vegetables

Purchasing fruits and vegetables while they are in season is hugely beneficial. Not only are they more affordable, but they're easier to find, and of course, fresher. It means that they haven't shipped as far, and also means fewer chemicals were needed to help them last in the wrong season.

Spring	Summer
Asparagus, cauliflower, new potatoes, broccoli, radishes, savoy cabbage, sorrel, spinach, spring greens, kale, broad beans, watercress, carrots, spring onions, rhubarb, greens.	Broad beans, broccoli, carrots, courgette, cucumbers, fennel, peas, garlic, green beans, lettuce, new potatoes, radishes, rocket, runner beans, salad onions, aubergines, beetroots, tomatoes, watercress, blueberries, plums, raspberries, strawberries.
Autumn	**Winter**
Beetroot, carrots, celeriac, field mushrooms, kale, leeks, marrow, potatoes, pumpkin, rocket, sorrel, squashes, sweetcorn, tomatoes. watercress, lettuce, apples, blackberries, damsons, elderberries, pears, plums.	Greens, beetroot, Brussels sprouts, cabbage, cauliflower, celeriac, chicory, fennel, Jerusalem artichokes, kale, chard, leeks, parsnips, potatoes, red cabbage, swede, turnips, apples, pears.

Stressed = Desserts

Keep In	Cut Out
Almond Milk	Alcohol
Apples	Barley
Apple Cider Vinegar	Biscuits
Artichoke	Borlotti Beans
Asparagus	Bread
Aubergine	Butter
Avocados	Caffeine
Bananas	Cakes
Beansprouts	Cereal
Beef	Cheese
Beetroot	Chocolate
Blackberries	Cookies
Blueberries	Crackers
Blue Cheese	Cream
Broccoli	Crème Fraiche
Brown Rice	Cream Cheese
Buckwheat	Desserts
Cabbage	Dried Fruit

Cannellini Beans	Fruit Juices
Cauliflower	Gluten
Carrots	Granola
Celeriac	Milk
Celery	Muesli Bars
Cherries	Pasta
Chicken	Rye
Chickpeas	Soft Drinks
Chicory	Sugar
Cocoa	Sweets
Coconut Cream	Wheat
Coconut Milk	White Rice
Coconut Water	Yoghurt
Courgette	
Cranberries	
Cucumber	
Duck	
Eggs	
Fennel	
Fruit Tea	
Garlic	
Goose	
Grapes	
Green Beans	

Haricot Beans	
Herbs (fresh)	
Herb tea	
Honey	
Kale	
Kidney Beans	
Kiwi	
Leeks	
Lemons	
Lettuce	
Lima Beans	
Lime	
Lychee	
Mange Tout	
Mango	
Melon	
Nuts	
Oats	
Olives	
Onions	
Oranges	
Pak Choy	
Papaya	
Peaches	

Pears

Peas

Peppers

Pineapple

Pomegranate

Pork

Pumpkin

Quinoa

Radish

Raspberries

Redcurrants

Roquefort

Seafood, especially oily fish such as salmon, mackerel, and sardines

Sea Weeds like nori, kelp, and dulse

Seeds

Spices (fresh)

Spinach

Squash

Strawberries

Stilton

Swede

Sweet Potatoes

Tamari

Tangerine	
Tomatoes	
Turkey	
Venison	
Water	
Water Chestnuts	

Bringing It All Together

The most obvious connection between clean living and your hair health is the impact that clean living has on your gut. We covered the power of a healthy gut on your body, mind, and hair pretty extensively in the last chapter, but it is important to note again that your hair growth relies on three things: blood flow, nutrients, and hormones. The nutrients come —in part—by how well your gut functions, but your gut can't send out nutrients that you aren't putting in. Enter, clean living. Clean living is your all-round guide for taking care of your body for peak performance. Eating fruits, veggies, protein, and healthy fats creates the much-needed balance.

Try This

Take a look back at the food log you created in chapter two. Get out your best red pen, and start making an X next to the foods that aren't a part of clean living. Use the "Cut It Out" list to help guide you. If you want to take it a step further, use the "Add In" list to find replacements for the food you are cutting out. For example, cross out that pasta and add in spaghetti courgette.

Now, it's time to make a plan. Armed with more information, make an initial plan for clean eating. Your plan will change as you learn more and become more comfortable with clean living.

Step One: Prepare your House!

1. Clean out your cupboard and your fridge of all no-no items (more on this in chapter five).

2. Using this chapter, make a list of staples that you can add in, such as spices, fruits, veggies, and proteins.

Step Two: Make a Menu!

You will not always require a menu to eat clean. However, when you are first getting started, it's important to have a set of meals planned out to fall back on. So, spend some time planning a week's worth of meals. Have your planner or calendar available while you start thinking about your meals. It's important to know how busy you will be on any given day, so you can leave more elaborate meals for the days where you don't have five meetings or three after-school drop-offs.

Chapter Four: SUGAR, OH HONEY, HONEY...

Chapter Four: SUGAR, OH HONEY, HONEY...

It's time to talk about sugar. You can't truly live or eat clean without tackling your sugar habit. You may be saying to yourself, 'But I don't have a sugar habit!' For some people that may be true, but in today's modern age of pre-packaged processed food and £5 sugar-laced lattes, hidden sugars are lurking everywhere. You might think you're having a healthy salad, but if you take a close look at the ingredient list on that salad dressing, I would be willing to bet there is sugar hiding somewhere on the label. I always pretended that I didn't have a sugar habit, because I was never one for cartons of fresh juice; however, I have been known to quash a few cans of Vanilla Coke in my time! And, that adds up.

According to government research, the average UK sugar intake is over the recommended health limit by about 11% for all age groups. This statistic isn't exactly shocking. Pre-packaged foods have been on the rise since we figured out how to produce, preserve, and ship uniform foods to the masses. These foods served their purpose during World War Two when they were used to feed troops, but since then, they have become a real danger to the overall health of the population. In order to take fresh foods and make them last long enough to ship and sit on shelves for weeks or even months, manufacturers load them up with preservatives—a process which removes a lot of the natural nutrients and flavour. To compensate for that, the companies pump the food with artificial flavours and sugars. Because sucrose is a preservative, and gives bulk as well as sweetness to certain foods, it is widely used in food processing.

When I say hidden sugar, that isn't a joke or an exaggeration. Companies have found all kinds of ways to disguise the sugar in your food with strange names. This is where my clean-living rule, of not eating anything with ingredients that I have never heard of, comes into play. Most of us know to look out for foods that list sugar as the first ingredient. But, more often than not, companies list sugar by two or three different names that you probably won't recognise. These are no longer listed first, because they are split up as "different" ingredients. Names include: sucrose, glucose, dextrose, maltose, molasses, lactose, fructose, honey, corn syrup, and invert syrup. There are at least **sixty-one** different names for sugar currently in use on food labels! If it's got an OSE at the end of it—it's sugar. That can of Vanilla Coke I mentioned has 42 grams of sugar! In the UK, it is recommended that adults shouldn't have more than 30 grams of sugar in a day. This just shows how easy it is to go over the recommended amount, and that's without even including the natural sugars you might eat in a day.

Added Sugar vs. Natural Sugar

It is important here to acknowledge the difference between added sugar and natural sugar. In pre-packaged products, you may never know if the food contains added or natural. This is because they purposefully don't distinguish the two. Your body is going to break down sugar in the same way, regardless of if it's natural sugar or added sugar. But, with regards to your health, there is a big difference.

Added sugar is highly processed and found in junk food. Natural sugars are found in a lot of natural foods, but are most commonly associated with fruit. So why is an apple good for you, but not that soda? The answer is simple. Fruit comes packed with loads of other nutrients, including vitamins, minerals, and fibre. All of these nourish your body and help you feel full and satisfied. Meanwhile, junk food consists almost entirely of empty calories, and has no benefits for your body.

Dangers of Sugar

While the NHS recommends no more than thirty grams of sugar per day, I suggest you cut out as much added sugar as possible. Added sugars provide no benefit to your body. Instead, they damage you, in both seen and unseen ways.

One of the first problems with sugar is that it goes one step beyond not satisfying your hunger. Instead, it leaves you hungrier than you were before you ate it! Sugar, like other "simple" grains, gets digested quickly, resulting in a fast rise of blood sugar levels. In response, your body releases a hormone called insulin, which in turn causes your blood sugar levels to drop equally as fast. We call this the "sugar crash" because when it's all over, you are left feeling tired, hungry, and irritable. Unfortunately, a lot of people reach for another dose of sugar to combat that feeling, only to restart the whole cycle again.

Aside from messing with our natural ability to detect hunger and keep ourselves balanced, sugar has been linked to a number of negative health effects. Too much sugar can contribute to weight gain, which of course is a health issue that comes with its own concerns. The list of negative effects of sugar on your body is extensive. It stresses the liver, weakens the immune system, increases bad cholesterol, and affects sleep. Sugar can also impact mental health, causing mood swings and increased risk of depression and anxiety.

On top of all this, sugar significantly increases your inflammation. If you remember from the "Gut Imbalance" section, inflammation in your gut means that your body cannot function at peak performance. By consuming sugar, you are actively working against your body's natural mechanisms to keep you healthy and balanced. Often, when people see their hair falling out or when they struggle to lose weight, they get angry at themselves or their body. They blame bad genetics, when the truth is that you are fighting a needless battle. Your body isn't your enemy!

Artificial Sweeteners

We talked about the dangers of sugar, but what about all those chemicals that make your sodas, cakes, and coffees sweet? First and foremost, these are a no-no when it comes to clean eating, for the simple fact that they are not natural. Remember, the goal of clean eating is to focus on natural, healthy options that will promote a balanced gut.

Artificial sweeteners (unlike sugar) aren't digested by your body at all. That doesn't mean, however, that they don't have to move through your gut. And, as they move through your gut, they have a significant impact. Studies have shown that artificial sweeteners affect the bacteria in the gut. In some cases, artificial sweeteners were found to kill off essential bacteria, while in others certain bacteria flourished, becoming overpopulated and imbalanced. Essentially, artificial sweeteners can re-wire the gut, often in dangerous and unhealthy ways. Overall the trend for the re-wired guts was toward obesity, glucose intolerance, and diabetes. So, while you might think you're making the healthier choice, you are really just substituting one unhealthy habit for another.

Cutting Out the Sweet Stuff

With all that being said, you'll be pleased to know that there is a relatively easy "fix." There are plenty of choices now that help when you are feeling "deprived" of your favourite treats. Yet, the truth is, breaking the sugar habit can be hard work. Packaged foods are convenient, and we have a lot of social conventions surrounding sugar, such as birthdays and holidays. And the other thing (of course) is...you might simply enjoy it! Sugar tastes good for a reason—it's designed to get you hooked. The sugar cycle can be a hard addiction to break for many people, who have become so used to the ups and downs. When they start to cut down on sugar or cut it out altogether, they suddenly feel dramatic crashes in energy, mood, and hunger. These can be heightened even more dramatically, because they don't have sugar to rescue them. We've all been there. Some days I am just so frickin' tired that I can't stop myself reaching for the chocolate. That is, of course, if it's in my cupboard in the first place! I now ration myself to two small chunks of chocolate only, when the fancy takes me. I know I could break that habit over twenty-eight days, but to be honest it's not such a bad one. A little of what you fancy does you good. After all, life is for living!

Breaking the sugar habit requires making small changes to your daily routine. First, you have to let go of guilt around food. In our "Diet with a capital D" culture, we are trained into thinking that food is either good or bad and that we should feel bad if we eat bad food. The problem with this kind of thinking is that it doesn't actually help us eat healthier. Instead, try to start thinking about your food as energy. When it gets dark outside, you turn on the lights. When your car is running low, you go to the petrol station. When your phone battery is dying, you charge it. When you are sick, you take medicine. You don't debate these things or feel guilty. The same should apply to food. Your food is your energy source. It keeps your body functioning. You don't need to feel guilty about fuelling your body, but you do need to be mindful about what your body needs vs what it doesn't.

> Eating an apple will fill you up, whereas drinking apple juice will make you fat.

Think of it this way: you wouldn't take antacid for a headache. Likewise, you also wouldn't take aspirin if you cut your finger. Similarly, if you want to feel energetic, stay awake through a presentation, or avoid losing your hair, you wouldn't (or shouldn't) feed your body fuel that is going to burn too fast and leave you tired, or fuel that will make you feel sick. When we get medicine from the doctor, most of us read the warning labels and side effects. Imagine if your food came with that too. Would you eat something if the packet told you that it may cause mood swings, depression, inflammation, weight gain, hormonal imbalance, increase in cholesterol, and insomnia? Given that there are NO known health benefits to sugar, it becomes a no brainer. All that is left is to retrain your thought process around sugar. Eating a piece of cake isn't a reward—it's a punishment.

Take a look at the log you made and your revisions from the past two "Try This" sections. Think about why the two food logs are so different. Was it simply because you didn't know any better? Or have you fallen into unhealthy patterns? Instead of reaching for that soda, opt for herbal tea, water (fizzy with lemon), lime juice, or just a slice of refreshing cucumber. Rather than mindlessly snacking on your child's leftover Halloween sweets, consider a piece of fruit, or a homemade treat. Start scrutinising these habits that have become so ingrained in your life. Ask yourself why you want that sugary snack. What benefit does it provide you, whether it is mental, emotional, social, or as a kick start at midday? Then, all you have to do is find an alternative that would fill that need.

For ideas on homemade treats visit "NutriHome" on my website, which is loaded with healthy ideas for you and your family members: https://simonethomaswellness.com/blogs/nutrihome

Bringing It All Together

Hopefully it isn't surprising to learn that sugar is really bad for your hair and skin. When you eat sugary foods, your blood sugar levels spike. As a response, your body releases insulin, whose job it is to allow your muscles, fat, and liver to absorb glucose. If we eat a lot of sugar, we have to also release a lot of insulin, and with that insulin release comes a release of androgen, a hormone that causes your hair follicles to shrink. Sugar also affects the way hormones and nutrients are processed and moved through the body, which means your hair isn't getting enough of what it needs.

Your skin will start showing signs of sugar damage pretty quickly too. Collagen, a protein we will talk about in chapter ten, plays a vital part in the health of your skin. When blood sugar goes up too rapidly, it can attach itself to collagen, stopping your skin getting any of this protein. Higher sugar levels also cause increased inflammation, which quickly shows in your skin. Lastly, too much sugar alters the very biochemical composition of your skin cells, causing them to age prematurely and lose elasticity.

Sarah, a 25-year-old client, came to me at Simone Thomas Salon because she was concerned about her thinning hair. Sarah suffered from Polycystic Ovary Syndrome, was overweight, had severe acne, and hadn't had a menstrual cycle for 10 months. I dove right in to start looking at her diet. I wasn't surprised to find that her diet looked like something that is becoming more and more typical: too few vegetables, fruits and protein, too much processed food and sugar. I prescribed a nutrition plan designed to tackle the insufficiencies in her current diet, alongside some of my Ginkgo Biloba B+ Supplements. Within three months, Sarah's periods had returned, her acne was clearing, she'd lost weight, and there was evidence of new hair growth. Sarah was blown away by the effect of her personalised diet, and the positive impact it had on her overall wellbeing.

Try This

If you are one of those people who have fallen prey to the sugar cycle of cravings, binges, crashes, and more cravings, then the first thing you need to do is make a commitment.

1. Clean out your cupboard (more on this in the next chapter).

2. Make small achievable goals. Depending on your individual situation, your goals are going to be different than someone else's. But, you want to set yourself up for success. So, think about what your

sugar triggers are. Do you crave sugar most after a stressful day? Maybe it is when you are bored or just sitting down to watch a movie? Maybe your goal, for the first day, is simply not to have a sweet after dinner or to avoid sugar in your morning coffee! Each day, the goals should grow and build until you have reached a larger one-month goal. Use the chart to create your goals.

My Sugar-Free Goals:

Day 1:	
Day 2:	
Day 3:	
Day 4:	
Day 5:	
Week 2:	
One Month:	

3. Make a plan for cravings. Spend time thinking about what you will do when you start craving sugar. Maybe you will reach for a healthy alternative (see next step), take a walk, or read through your goals.

4. Have healthy alternatives handy. If you start getting sugar cravings, don't rely on willpower alone to get you through it. I have included some healthy alternatives to sugar-filled treats that you can grab and go without feeling like you are depriving yourself or falling off the wagon! Carve out an hour over the weekend prepping some healthy alternatives, so you have them all week.

5. Eat more often. Remember, going too long between meals and letting yourself get too hungry will lead your body to think it's starving. And when your body has convinced itself that it's starving, you will get sugar cravings big time!

Use the chart on the next page to help you analyse and revise your sugar cravings.

Craving. Describe when the craving hit, what it was for, and what was happening at the time.	Trigger. What do you think triggered the craving? What need would sugar have filled? (Think: emotional, social, stress relief, over-hungry etc.)	Alternative. What can you eat or do instead, to distract from the craving? (Think: eat a healthy snack, go for a walk, revisit your goals.)

Chapter Five: CUPBOARD LOVE

There is only one of you—you are unique.

How often do you feel as though you are running on empty? So many of us walk through life in a mild haze, struggling to keep our energy levels up enough to accomplish only the most basic agendas. At times when I go out with my boys, I often do so without a crumb of food in my stomach. I have my bag loaded with snacks for the kids, but of course nothing for myself. So, it's no surprise that my mood is also low, my patience with the boys runs extraordinarily thin, and any level of self-esteem or happiness is, generally speaking, sucked right out of me. It's all fine and well to talk about eating healthier, cutting out sugar and processed food, and bringing your gut health back to life, but it is another thing to follow through.

So, how do you find your way back when life is chaotic, unpredictable, and often exhausting? It starts with a clear and practical plan. It isn't enough to simply decide you will eat clean—you have to make a plan to back it up. We have been slowly building your plan over the last few chapters. A clean eating plan begins with recognising what constitutes healthy, clean living, and what roadblocks have historically prevented you from making those choices. The next step is getting organised.

Time to Get Organised

I truly believe that, first and foremost, you have to be organised in order to meet your clean eating goals. Getting organised means setting yourself up for success. This ensures that when you hit a roadblock, have a long day at work, or find yourself starving midday, you aren't reaching for junk food or getting cranky with everyone around you.

Part of that plan is thinking about what you will keep in your cupboard. Is your cupboard filled with junk food for the kids? Is it empty more often than not? Is it filled with fancy ingredients to make elaborate meals? Regardless of what your cupboard looks like right now, you probably aren't spending enough time getting it organised. You've got to treat your food cupboard as another member of your family, and pay it equal attention. Set aside time every week to ensure that you give your cupboard the care it deserves. When I did this, I not only became happier and healthier, but I was a far better person to be around. In the end, your ability to follow a healthy eating plan stems from your cupboard and your fridge, and what's in them. I set aside some time each week to go through my cupboard and fridge, to clean them out and make sure they are well stocked with all the essential "good for me" foods.

First comes the clean-out. Go through your cupboard with a bin bag in hand. Be ruthless! If the items in there either never get used or don't serve your goal, get rid of them. I am sure many of you have kids and you are saying to yourself, 'How will my kids survive without crisps, cookies, and sugary yoghurts?' It may be tough, but training them now to eat healthy, nutritious snacks means they won't have to re-train themselves later, like you are doing.

Next comes refilling your cupboard. Filling your cupboard comes in three parts: healthy "go-to" snacks, everyday staples, and fresh items.

Healthy "Go-To" Snacks

Ensure that your cupboard is ALWAYS full and primed up with easy "go-to" snacks (all of the healthy option variety), and you will find your way back to happiness surprisingly quickly. Not only will you feel in control, but you will get an enormous feeling of satisfaction!

Think about the different types of foods you snack on. Sometimes you crave something crunchy, other times you are looking for something sweet, or maybe you like salty. Regardless of your preferences, you can find a healthy, natural, CLEAN alternative. Spend some time in the "Try This" section of this chapter filling out the suggested lists. You will find that there are several healthier alternatives to your regular snacks. It is important to keep all of these things to hand, so when you are rushing out the door or late in making dinner, you don't reach for a cookie instead of something healthier.

Remember, clean eating is not a calorie-cutting diet. You should never be starving or depriving yourself of food. When you consume too few calories or go too long between meals, the consequences are similar to a sugar crash and an unhealthy diet. Essentially, your body goes into starvation mode. This causes your blood sugar levels to crash, your metabolism to slow, and your muscles to break down.

All of this is to say, you need to eat! The point of clean living is to nourish your body, not to starve it. Don't be afraid of snacks or carbs or fats, as long as they are clean, healthy alternatives. Make sure you have all kinds of snacks, but most importantly, keep quick, easy snacks for those times when you can't bake healthy cookies from scratch.

Nowhere in this book will I talk about calorie counting, but what I will do is differentiate between good and bad foods. Ultimately, the choice is yours. Basically, if it's covered in metal or plastic—forget it.

> There are too many people counting calories and not enough people counting chemicals.

Choose nutritious light bites and snacks. I always have carrot and cucumber crudité in the fridge, which I dip into guacamole or humous—the more garlicky the better! Check out "NutriHome" for recipes and snack ideas!

I also have a big jar of unsalted nuts—a handful of almonds, Brazil nuts, or raw cashews works wonders for keeping the hunger pangs away—and if I fancy something sweet then I'll opt for a treat with my homemade banana bread, which I keep in a tin for longevity.

The alternatives are out there, so long as you take the time to look for them!

Everyday Staples

Now it's time to focus on your main meals. Regardless of the types of food you like to eat or cook, chances are you spend your time at the supermarket picking up the same things time and time again. 60% of us eat the same meals every week, and don't have much diversity to what we're cooking each month. That being said, everyday staples are important, and the same is true for clean eating. There will be certain cupboard foods that you need all the time. Everyday staples stem from the ingredients that you find in many of your meals.

Understanding and stocking up on your everyday staples is key to organising and to the success of clean living. Too often, people jump into a new "diet" or lifestyle and try to re-write every habit all at once, doing away with their old favourite meals and replacing them with elaborate alternatives, filled with exotic ingredients that you have to hunt for in the grocery store. Unfortunately, these kinds of total re-writes aren't sustainable. Eventually, you will burn out, whether in a week or a month, and you will find yourself falling back into familiar easier habits. The solution is to keep it easy! Keep your kitchen filled with all of your staples that you are familiar with, so long as they meet the clean-living standards. Look at your list from chapter three's "Try This". What can you keep in your diet? What can you modify to fit into clean living? For instance, if you eat instant oatmeal every morning, maybe you can make overnight oats filled with fresh fruit that you keep in your fridge for two days.

Start each week by developing a menu. Within that menu, include some easy meals, which can be made in under thirty minutes, and that only revolve around staples. I have developed a lot of thirty-minute meals that I share on NutriHome (via my website). Once you have your menu, make your "staples" grocery list. This list is just the things that you need ALL of the time. We will add in the fresh produce and occasional items in the next section. By focusing just on the things you need regularly, you can keep a running list that you simply check off or uncheck. In fact, I get food delivered twice a week: one large delivery and one top up (for the fresh stuff). A big thank you to Abel & Cole, and Waitrose, for this!

We're all familiar with the feeling of getting home after a really busy day, opening the fridge, and not finding anything to eat. That is a bad situation on a normal day, but when you are trying to eat clean for the first time, it can be extremely detrimental. There's nothing that helps to create a smooth cooking experience more than prepping your ingredients before you start. Doing this helps to ensure you don't get halfway through your recipe before realising you are missing an ingredient. I've noticed that when everything is prepped and ready to go, a calm is created in the kitchen, and this allows me to savour and enjoy what I'm doing.

The Fresh Stuff

By "fresh stuff", I am of course referring to ingredients that may be specific to a certain recipe, or the ingredients that can't live in your cupboard for a week at a time—think fruits, vegetables, fresh meats, and seafood. You are going to organise and plan for these things in the same way you did your snacks and everyday staples. But, this time, you will need a little more planning.

Again, spend some time each week thinking about the meals you want for the week. What fruits, vegetables, and meats are needed? What fruits and veggies can you fit into your breakfast, lunch, and snacks? Develop your list and plan to replenish those items twice a week. Delivery boxes can be a huge help here. While my meat and fish are from the local butchers and fishmongers, I subscribe to a weekly vegetable box from Abel & Cole, who are an organic food delivery company. Every Thursday, anything from eight boxes or more arrives with me, full of amazing fruits, vegetables, house staples, and sometimes even a heavenly crumble and custard treat!

Love What You Eat

Loving what you eat follows directly on. Be honest, did you cringe at the words "clean living", assuming you had to eat kale smoothies, and cut out all flavour? Seriously now—if it's in a jar or in a packet, it's processed more often than not. If you are a sixties, seventies, or eighties baby like me, you were most probably brought up on the wonderful new invention of ready meals and tv dinners i.e. processed food. And yes, you developed a taste for it, citing food unflavoured and untampered with as bland. But an amazing thing happens when you start eating clean, cutting out excess salt, chemicals, and sugar: your taste buds change. You find the subtleties of the different flavours and spices in your food.

So, you don't have to hate your food, you don't have to eat salads every day, and you don't have to fill your cupboard with rice cakes and bland, flavourless "health foods". You can fill your cupboards with *whatever you want*! You can love what you eat. It is just a matter of retraining, organising, and preparing.

Fortunately for me, when I was a child my mum cooked everything from scratch. But it wasn't to enhance my wellbeing—her nickname amongst friends and family was "salmonella"; she was famous for her dinosaur leg curry. Nothing went to waste, believe me. This trait has remained in the family, as my brother now does it too. Both my boys have had very little processed food, nor will they be encouraged to. The amount of processed food that can be found on the table when they dine with their fellow lunch dates alarms me. Is there really any need for a three-year-old to tuck into a chocolate-covered mini roll washed down with a carton of fruit juice? What's wrong with fresh fruit or crudité for a snack? My boys really do make happy noises when they find grapes, strawberries, or blueberries in their lunch box—they love them. Ashton is broccoli mad!

If you are a family that already cooks your meals at home, then your task here is easier. Simply start replacing pre-packaged ingredients with fresh ones. Plan your meals around the clean eating guidelines. If your family does not cook meals at home and relies heavily on pre-packaged snacks and meals, then it can be overwhelming to change these habits. Take heart that you have already begun, simply by reading this book and educating yourself. Take each step one at a time. You can start by simply cooking more meals at home. Ready-made and takeaway foods are usually packed with chemicals, salt, sugar, and fat. When cooking, you can make larger batches and freeze them in individual portions to create your own "ready meals". That way you can control what you're eating and the portion size, making sure it is filled with whole grains, lean protein, fresh fruits, and vegetables, while still having a "ready to go" meal when it's late and you are busy.

If you are daunted by the idea of tossing all the sweets and junk in the bin—remember, if it's not in the house, you can't eat it! There may be times when you crave that candy bar or cookie, but you will have to find an alternative when you have removed those temptations. Children will follow suit too. It is hard to imagine your picky eater sitting down to a plate of raw veggies and enjoying themselves, but if you don't give them the chance, they will never be able to develop a liking for them.

Making the Swap

Swapping out the good for the bad doesn't have to be an overly difficult task. The more you do it, the easier it will become, until it's something you don't have to think about at all! Don't be put off if you don't have the exact ingredients that a new recipe may call for. As your confidence grows, you will find it far more satisfying to add your own twist to basic recipes!

Here is a quick cheat sheet for the most common swaps:

Sugar

Swap sugar for sweeteners such as cinnamon, maple syrup, raw honey, molasses, or dates. Dates are very sweet, but also full of nutrients. Soften them in boiling water, then grind them up in a food processor or blender, before adding them to sauces, dressings, and drinks.

Soda

Swap out soft drinks. As we covered earlier, these contain extremely high levels of added sugar. Diet drinks are often sweetened with aspartame, an artificial sweetener. Instead, drink water or naturally flavoured teas such as green, matcha, or herbal teas. You can also infuse sparkling water with any fresh fruit you have to hand.

Salt

Salt is one of those foods that you have to work on minimising. We often get way too much salt without even realising. Himalayan pink salt is toxin-free and full of minerals. You can also add this to your bathwater, to help release toxins.

Pasta, White Bread, White Rice

Pasta, white bread, and white rice have all been processed to the point of being unrecognisable from their source ingredients. Luckily, we now have lots of readily available healthy grains that can replace them, which is especially useful when you're looking for healthy carbs to balance out a meal. Try nutrient-rich quinoa instead.

Oil

Rather than spraying pans with chemicals or loading up on greasy unhealthy fats, cook with healthy oils, such as unrefined, cold-pressed coconut oil or extra virgin olive oil. My favourite is Lucy Bee.

Milk

Milk's a funny one. Humans are the only species that consume the milk of another animal, and the only species that intentionally drink milk past childhood. It's not surprising that we find it hard to tolerate, and that it can have an untoward effect on the body. In fact, many people have some level of dairy and lactose intolerance that they aren't even aware of. Today there are many variants available to us other than cow's milk. We are a lactose-free household, and thoroughly enjoy almond milk—it also works to feed the skin, helping you to feel full, thanks to the fibre content. You can, of course, buy almond milk in the store, but be sure to read the labels and make sure they haven't snuck in any sugar! Or, if you are like me, you can make your own. I do this by using an amazing machine, called "Almond Cow", which is a plant-based milk maker. Alternatively, consider cashew or coconut milk. Beware of rice milk, as it is very sugary, and oat milk can contain small traces of gluten. I always opt for a dairy-free choice for cooking and yoghurts. My favourite dairy-free yoghurt is the Coconut Collaborative.

> If you eat shit, you'll look and feel like shit.

Bringing It All Together

"Cupboard Love" is all about setting yourself up for success. We can read all the books on healthy eating, or use all the latest hair care products for perfect tresses, but if we don't set ourselves up for success then we certainly won't find any. It is all too easy to fall back into the old patterns that have sustained us for most of our lives, and much harder to find ways to break the cycle. As you start cleaning out your cupboards, keep your goals in mind. Why are you doing this? What does success look like for you? Is it healthier hair? A more attractive appearance? More energy? Regardless of your reason, keep that in mind as you start clearing out the cupboard, and be honest about your ingrained bad habits.

Crash "diets" can be just as bad for your health and hair as eating junk every day. So, don't keep those cookies around for a "bad" day or because the kids like them so much. Focus your efforts on a lifestyle change, not a temporary quick fix. Eating a clean diet for a month is great, but if you let yourself fall back into unhealthy habits then your hair will show it!

Try This

By the end of this section, you will have planned out your meals for a week, snack alternatives, and two "ready-to-shop" grocery lists. Before we get there though, I want to share with you what the meals for my day look like. If you are brand new to clean eating, you may not even know what kinds of foods to eat. When we get to your turn, you can simply copy my meals (if that works best for you) but don't be afraid to start playing around with what you like and finding new recipes.

The Way I Do It

Simone's morning routine:

Hot water and lemon juice—BUT DON'T PUT THE LEMON IN THE WATER! Pesticides and chemicals stay on the skin of the lemon. When you put a slice in your hot water, those chemicals seep off the skin and into your water, until you are drinking things you don't want to be drinking.

We have touched upon the importance of supplements to help the vitamin and mineral deficiencies you may have in your diet. I use my own brand "Simone Thomas Wellness" from www.simonethomaswellness.com. You can use another brand of supplements, but mine are specifically formulated to include everything we have talked about in this book, and for hair, nails, gut health, and overall wellbeing.

The supplements I rely on:

- 2 x Everyday Wellbeing tablets.

- 2 x Super Green Capsules. 2 x Biotin Capsules. There is also a Gingko Capsule available for those focused more on hair loss. I swap to these in winter months when our hair is more prone to shredding/there's more chance of a disrupted hair growth cycle.

This is the same routine Jessica Wright takes for her Simone Thomas Wellness routine. Find out more about Jessica here: https://simonethomaswellness.com/blogs/news/how-jessica-wright-improved-her-health-with-simone-thomas-wellness-supplements

My Breakfast

For breakfast, I focus on protein. Protein provides the long-lasting energy I need throughout the day. This takes the form of overnight oats, omelettes, or dairy-free yoghurts with fruit. For a change or at weekends I opt for protein and fat intake for muscle growth and repair. I make a lovely smoked kipper breakfast muffin, which I eat with a sprinkling of black pepper.

My Lunch

I toss together sliced asparagus (quick boiled and cooled), red pepper, tomatoes, mixed leaves, broccoli, avocado, olives, and quinoa in a large bowl and scatter seeds (any seeds work here. I opt for any seed or nut mix that I have around) and mint on top for flavour. This goes into my fridge, and I can help myself and take out portions throughout the course of the next few days, which I transfer to my lunchbox. I also make a lime and chilli dressing, which I keep in a screw-top jar in the fridge and pour on the salad just before eating. I don't recommend storing foods in the fridge for longer than two days (as this leads to bacterial growth). The gut also needs diversity, so you should avoid eating the same meal more than twice a week anyway.

> Turn off all distractions, sit down, eat slowly. Eat until you are satisfied, not until you are stuffed.

My Dinner

For dinner, I really do like to mix it up, as I enjoy cooking at night. In the colder months, I make more warm meals like home-made soups and casseroles. The open fire goes on and I listen to music while I cook. I might make a home-made sauce, which could be garlic, rosemary, chopped tomatoes, lemon, sea salt, and a drizzle of olive oil, then add chicken which has been marinating in the fridge for twenty-four hours beforehand. I'd serve this with asparagus and other green vegetables, or in the summer, feta salad with mixed seeds. My other favourites are marinated white fish with Cajun spices served with sweet potato and broccoli, or Thai red chicken curry with rice. If I have energy and am feeling extra good then I will make a cauliflower rice. Soup-wise, I make vegetable soup or a mixed mushroom soup (I try to add four different types of mushrooms). I call this "the magic mushroom soup", as it boosts the immune system.

In the summer I often go with salmon, with a mixed salad bowl made of beansprouts, aubergine, cucumber, sesame seeds, and a dressing. Alternatively, I might just have chicken and home-made slaw salad. I also have my super greens and "Everyday Wellbeing" in a night-time plant protein drink, with unsweetened almond milk and maybe a mix of fruits as well. I always try to follow an anti-inflammatory diet as much as possible, and for me a Mediterranean diet makes me feel at my best.

Now it is your turn!

Let's start with snacks—I want to make it as easy as possible for you to transition to clean living. Take a look at the list you made in chapter two of "Cut-out and Add-Ins". Fill out the chart with the types of snack foods you crave—this can be actual foods like crisps and cookies, or it can be categories of foods like sweet, savoury, or crunchy. Once you have that list filled out, write down several options for healthy, clean replacements (both "quick" and "slow") that can be prepped ahead of time. I made a sample chart to get you started, but remember you should love what you eat, so don't force yourself to eat my suggestions. Instead, come up with your own alternatives that meet your needs.

Craving	Replacement Options (Quick)	Replacement Options (Slow)
Sweet		
Savoury		
Crunchy		
Cookies and Cakes		

Craving	Replacement Options (Quick)	Replacement Options (Slow)

Now let's do the same thing for our everyday staples. Run through your day's meals, and for each type of meal write down the ingredients that you use at least once or twice a week (that don't go bad). Remember these are not the fresh foods, so you might use tomatoes every day, but you can't order them once and have them still be fresh days later. If you are serious about eating clean, then take the time to fill this chart out, even if you *think* you know what your go-to staples are. Getting yourself organised is a huge part of sticking to a new plan. This will also help make sure none of the things in your shopping basket go against the clean-living rules.

Meal	Common Ingredients
Breakfast	
Lunch	
Dinner	
Snacks	

From this list, create a "Master Shopping List". When you go to the super-market, you can make smaller, more specific shopping lists, based on your master shopping list.

Now it's time to do the same thing with your fresh ingredients. This list will also include any specialised ingredients that you need just for one meal, but that you may not use all the time. So, this list will likely change, but the fresh products probably won't. Again, making a master list saves you time, money, and keeps you on track—so don't skip this step.

Chapter Six: WATER WORKS

The most common mistake I notice with my clients is that they don't drink enough water. And yet, water is the only drink that doesn't contain any sugar, calories, or additives. You should ALWAYS have a bottle of water with you throughout the day to keep hydrated. You will have heard it before, but I am going to say it again: you cannot be healthy without water! We all need to drink at least 2 litres (8 glasses) of water daily to hydrate our bodies, our brain, and our gut. Water plays a huge role in our overall health.

The Facts

The Stomach

The stomach needs water in two important ways, both of which are related to hydrochloric acid.

First, water is required to produce hydrochloric acid at the proper pH levels. Although water is not actually in the stomach at the same time as the hydrochloric acid, it's in the body when the hydrochloric acid is created, and promotes the proper pH level. When the contents of the stomach are not acidic enough, a little valve called the pylorus fails to open. Thus, the contents of the stomach don't pass into the duodenum. This is when dehydration occurs. The stomach really wants to get rid of its contents, so it tries moving them in the other direction—up into the oesophagus. However, the stomach's contents are still acidic. So, that acid burns the oesophagus, which results in heartburn. Think of all the pharmaceutical drugs for heartburn and indigestion that could be eliminated just by drinking enough water!

The pH of the acid in your stomach must be the right level for digestion to start, but that perfect pH alone is too acidic for the tissue of the stomach itself. This brings us to the second important function of water in the stomach. To protect itself, the stomach lining produces mucus, without which the acid comes into direct contact with the stomach tissue. This results in stomach ulcers. When we are dehydrated, the stomach doesn't have enough fluids to produce the mucus.

Blood Circulation

Even mild dehydration can affect your blood circulation and cardiovascular system. Not drinking enough water can increase your heart rate, decrease cardiac output, increase blood pressure, and cause orthostatic hypotension. While your cardiovascular system is a complex network, when it doesn't have enough water, it can't contract and restrict properly. This causes your heart to work harder for less output and your veins to have less elasticity. Orthostatic hypotension means that when you stand up too quickly you feel dizzy and lightheaded, because your blood volume becomes too low for your body to adjust to the change in position.

Kidney Health

Your kidneys are responsible for removing the toxins and waste from your system—so they perform a pretty important task. When you become dehydrated, your kidneys can't get the nutrients they need to function at top performance. This is because your blood isn't moving so well. Even mild dehydration, if frequent enough, can lead to permanent kidney damage. Not getting enough water can also cause a build-up of waste and acids which hurt the kidneys even more. You will also be more prone to kidney stones!

Lymphatic System

Your lymphatic system is tied closely to your immune system and cardiovascular systems, and is responsible for removing harmful bacteria and viruses. Just like the cardiovascular system, when you aren't drinking enough fluids, your body can't move your blood as effectively as it should. When the lymphatic system slows down, that means it can't remove bacteria and viruses, which in turn means you will get sicker. My bi-weekly treat to myself is a ninety-minute full body lymphatic and toning massage, with an incredible therapist.

Balance Bodily Fluids

Drinking water also helps to maintain the balance of body fluids. Our bodies are 60% water, and the functions of these bodily fluids include digestion, absorption, circulation, creation of saliva, transportation of nutrients, and maintenance of body temperature.

Skin, Hair, and Nail Health

Without enough water, your skin, hair, and nails are the first to suffer. In dehydrated people, the fluid is being redirected to more vital functions, which means the skin, hair, and nails will dry out quicker, as they are receiving fewer nutrients. Some studies have even linked hair loss to dehydration.

Temperature Regulation

Water itself holds its temperature longer than the air. So, the more fluid we have in our body, the more we are able to regulate our own temperature when exercising, or when it's too hot/too cold.

Joint Health

Your joints need proper blood volume, in order to cushion movement. When you don't have enough water intake in a day, your blood volume level is lower, which puts more pressure on the joints. Over time, this can cause damage to said joints.

In conclusion, we can see that water is necessary for your body to function, as it plays a vital role in digestion, blood circulation, and skin health, as well as helping your body absorb nutrients and eliminate toxins. It can be so easy to not drink enough—one in five people drink less than the recommended daily intake. All of the clean eating in the world won't help if you aren't getting enough water!

Subtle Signs of Dehydration

When we think of dehydration, we often think of people in the movies struggling through the desert on the brink of death. The truth is, your body will let you know way before that point, with both subtle and not-so-subtle warnings. All you have to do is pay attention and know what to look out for.

- Infrequent urination or only urinating small amounts each time you go.

- Dark yellow urination—urine should be clear or as close to clear as possible.

- Dry skin or cracked lips.

- Sunken eyes.

- Few or no tears.

- Dry mouth.

- Constipation.

- Muscle cramping.

- Anxiety.

- Depression.

Stay Hydrated

Here are some tips for staying hydrated throughout the day.

- Start every day, as I do, with a glass of hot water and lemon. This helps to flush out impurities that have been processed overnight.

- Keep a large bottle or jug with you and sip from it throughout the day. This will keep you energised and your skin nourished, which in turn will help to reduce the appearance of fine lines.

- Your body is mildly dehydrated after sleep, so make sure that you drink a glass of water first thing in the morning. This also helps your body flush out toxins before your first meal, keeps your skin supple and radiant, and boosts your energy for the day ahead—reducing the temptation to snack unnecessarily!

- If you feel thirsty, it's a sign that your body has been craving water for some time. Take small drinks often, and don't wait to feel thirsty before drinking.

- The hormones that trigger hunger and thirst are the same, which means that you can mistake long-lasting thirst for hunger. Next time you feel a hunger pang, try drinking a glass of water instead of reaching for a snack.

- Drink a glass of water before each meal. This habit will help prevent overeating and will also prepare your stomach for digestion.

- Alcohol is a diuretic that causes your kidneys to produce large quantities of urine, depleting the body of skin-nourishing nutrients and drying it out. Drinking just one alcoholic drink can cause your body to lose a disproportionally large quantity of liquid, and the effects continue even after you've stopped drinking. So, if you are drinking alcohol, drink twice as much water as you normally would.

- Make sure you're hydrated before going to sleep. This keeps your skin nourished during the night. Drink a glass of water shortly before going to bed. Night time is usually the longest period your body will go without a drink, so it's important that your hydration levels are topped up beforehand. My award-winning "SkinQuencher" is my nightly go-to, containing hydrolysed marine collagen and vitamin C. Marine collagen is known to be easily absorbed by the body and is renowned for its ability to heal, regenerate, and repair. Vitamin C contributes to normal collagen formation for the normal function of blood vessels, bones, cartilage, gums, skin, and teeth.

- Marine collagen is known to be easily absorbed by the body and is renowned for its ability to heal, regenerate and repair. Vitamin C contributes to normal collagen formation for the normal function of blood vessels, bones, cartilage, gums, skin, and teeth.

- Buy yourself a reusable bottle—mine is fantastic, and I wouldn't be without it. I love the fact that if it had the chance to hold water for twenty-four hours (it doesn't, as I am drinking all the time) it would still be as cold as it was when I filled the bottle. Likewise, it keeps the temperature hot for twelve hours if you want a hot drink.

Bringing It All Together

Dehydration is the second most damaging thing you can do to your skin, second only to poor diet. When your body loses more water than it is taking in, you become dehydrated. When your body is dehydrated, your skin will show it first. This is because your body is pulling that much-needed water from your skin to make sure your blood continues to flow, and to keep your organs functioning. Without enough water in your body, your skin can no longer regulate body temperature or hold its elasticity. This is where premature fine lines and wrinkles come in.

Dehydration can also lead to hair loss and breakage. One quarter of your hair's make up consists of water. This means that without enough water, you cannot grow new hair. Thus, the existing hair you have becomes brittle and breaks more easily. Getting enough water can also help with dry scalp and dandruff. So, supple skin and glossy hair may be a simple glass of water away! While not getting enough water may be the cause of some of the most immediate and drastic effects on hair and skin, it's an easy fix.

Try This

Set a water goal for yourself. Once you make your daily goal, think about when you will drink your water. You don't want to get to 8:00 p.m. and realise you still have six glasses of water to drink. Rather than leaving it to chance, make yourself mini-goals. When will you drink each glass? How much will you have had by certain times in the day? Drinking water isn't rocket science. In fact, it is probably one of the easiest recommendations in this book, and yet we don't do it! The only way to change that is to make a conscious effort and a plan!

7AM:_____

8AM:_____

9AM:_____

10AM:_____

11AM:_____

12AM: _____

1PM: _____

2PM:_____

3PM:_____

4PM:_____

5PM:_____

6PM:_____

7PM:_____

8PM:_____

9PM:_____

Eat Your Water!

In addition to drinking your eight glasses of water, you can also *eat* your water. A lot of foods have crazily high-water content that helps you get your nutrients and keeps you hydrated.

Eat water...	
Red pepper	92% water
Tomatoes	94% water
Broccoli	91% water
Celery	95% water
Watermelon	92% water
Grapefruit	91% water

Chapter Seven: WELL BE ME

Alright, we have talked about what you are putting into your body and how it is either helping or hurting you. Now, it's time to talk about what you are doing with your body. It is really hard to be healthy without being active. It is true that as far as a healthy weight is concerned, about 80% depends on what you eat and 20% depends on the exercise you do, but those numbers don't address your overall health. (Not to mention, we can't simply ignore that 20% either.)

Recent studies have found that not getting enough cardio can be riskier and cause more damage to your body and overall health than smoking! In his study, Dr Wael Jaber found that being unfit in a stress test had a worse prognosis than that of diabetes, hypertension, and smoking. "It should be treated almost as a disease that has a prescription, which is called exercise," he said.

We have always known that exercise is important. Overall, getting regular exercise keeps you physically fit, which makes just about everything in life easier, from bringing in the groceries to taking the dog for a walk, to playing with the kids or keeping up at the office. It helps our cardiovascular system, heart health, and can help maintain a healthy weight. But now we understand that not getting exercise can actually be damaging to our long-term health, it's time to commit to moving your body. My weekly go-to and recommendation to my clients, is to follow "Brooke Burke Body" for the ultimate carved and contoured female body. For those who like to push themselves, follow Joe Wicks and Courtney Black, both of whom will get you sweating just with the warmup! As a bonus to improving your overall health, you are also going to see some of these amazing extra benefits:

The Transfer Effect

Turns out there is a hidden benefit to exercising—it leads you to eating healthily! Studies have found that people who exercise regularly, eat healthier. While this may seem like a conscious choice, it turns out that when you learn one new habit, it triggers you to learn and adopt other similar habits.

Boost Metabolism

Your metabolism is the chemical reaction of your body turning food into energy. A high metabolism means that you burn calories faster and can therefore eat more without gaining weight. When you build your muscles through exercise, your metabolism speeds up, even when you aren't exercising. Muscles need and use more calories than fat cells, so when you have more muscles, you metabolise more calories in a shorter amount of time.

Better Sleep

This one is pretty self-explanatory. When you tire out your body physically, you will sleep better. Regular exercise helps both the length and quality of your sleep.

Fight Depression

Exercise releases a few chemicals: catecholamines, endorphins, and dopamine. Catecholamines and endorphins are hormones that instantly lighten your mood, help you focus, and reduce pain. Dopamine essentially sends messages around in your brain, telling it to be happy.

Stronger Bones

We don't often think of our bones as a living part of our bodies in the same way we think of our muscles, but our bones *are* made of living tissue that grows and changes in similar ways. After the age of twenty, our bones stop growing naturally, but with exercise we can keep building bone strength and density. This is vital for our health, since bones store calcium, support our muscles, protect our organs, and provide a frame for our bodies. Muscles are important, but without healthy bones, your mobility will decline significantly as you age.

Longer Life

If everything I mentioned so far isn't enough to get you up and moving, then let me throw some stats at you:

- Women with low fitness levels have a higher risk of dying from a number of causes, including cardiac arrest, coronary artery disease, heart failure, stroke, and even cancer.

- Men with low fitness levels have a threefold greater risk for cardiovascular disease mortality, compared with high-fitness men.

It's simple, really. Even light exercise can improve your overall health, seriously lower your risk of death, and extend your life!

Finding a Balance

When I first embarked on an exercise routine, I went hell for leather, jumping in feet-first to intensive and frequent exercise. I quickly learned that this was a mistake. I had put my body under far too much stress, and caused my adrenals to release more cortisol, which in turn was bad for my gut! In essence, I'd reversed all the good that the exercise was meant to achieve.

So, what does this mean for you? You don't have to push yourself to exhaustion to reap the benefits of exercise! I have found that people fall into one of two categories. They either push too hard, too fast, and burn themselves out, or they find themselves making endless excuses about being too busy or not having the money to pay for a gym membership.

I am here to say, exercise can be easy! And most importantly, it should fit into YOUR lifestyle. You don't have to be like those Instagram stars to get healthy. I've found walking, boxing, swimming, pilates, and weightlifting to be my most mentally exhilarating exercises. I also grab the opportunity to walk outdoors as often as I can. Walking outdoors actually allows us to feel peaceful, and is far more relaxing than thinking about a physical routine at the gym. Studies have actually found that exercising outdoors left people feeling more revitalised and energetic than exercising inside.

Most self-help books are all about taking a walk in your lunch hour. Sadly, not everyone gets one (including me). So, in order to get my twenty-minute walk on a particularly hectic day, I park as far away as possible from my office and walk—returning to the car at the end of the day. Generally speaking, by the time I've done this walk, my head has totally cleared of my day's activities and I drive home feeling refreshed.

So, to summarise, you don't have to invest in expensive equipment or gym fees to make exercise a part of your life. There are plenty of different forms of activity that can be built into your routine. Fitting in more physical activity is not about burning the greatest number of calories in the shortest amount of time. Instead, it is about achieving a clean lifestyle. Your goal is to get your heart rate up for at least twenty to thirty minutes a day.

Exercise Tips to Get You Started

Water

We just had a whole chapter on how important water is, but it is even more important when you are exercising. Drink plenty of liquids before and during exercise in order to stay hydrated and keep your skin glowing. Your body can lose up to one litre of water per hour during exercise through sweating. Be careful not to drink too much just after you've finished exercising, as this may cause your muscles to cramp!

Walking

When walking, aim for ten or fifteen minutes a day to start off with. Your goal should be to build up to at least thirty minutes within a few weeks. Swing your arms and walk fast enough to work up a slight sweat; you should be slightly out of breath. Don't fall into the trap of thinking that walking isn't a good form of exercise. With the fitness blogging industry and boutique gyms showing muscled bodies drenched in sweat, it is all too easy to assume that if you aren't falling on your face after your workout, you aren't working out at all. Like I said at the start, it is possible to work too hard! But beyond that, walking is great for you! If it was all you could fit in, then you would still be well on your way to a healthier you! Walking boasts all the benefits of other types of exercise, without the added stress to your joints and muscles that higher impact exercises might have.

Jogging

If you feel ready for something a little more intense and higher impact, you can add in some jogging. If you are brand new to jogging, start by getting the right shoes! I know, it sounds vain, but it isn't. Not all shoes can withstand the strain of jogging. Try adding some short jogs into your walk. If you are walking for twenty minutes, add one-minute intervals of walking and jogging right in the middle, to total six minutes. Each time you go out for a walk, you can increase your intervals. Gradually build up your speed, distance, and the number of times a week that you go jogging. Don't overdo it. If you listen to your body, you will know what's working and what isn't.

Swimming

The wonderful thing about swimming is that you can get a good workout without any stress on your joints or bones. When you are submerged in water even only up to your waist, the water holds about 50% of your body weight. That means that while you are still getting your heart rate up, you aren't putting a strain on your body. For every ten minutes of intense swimming, you are burning one hundred and fifty calories. If you're doing the backstroke, you are still burning eighty calories every ten minutes! If you get bored swimming up and down, or if you cannot swim at all, consider trying some pool exercises or join an aqua-aerobics class. Swimming and water exercise are good complementary activities. If you are lucky enough to live by the sea, like I do, then try cold water swimming. This is something I have got into since 2020 and lockdown. My body feels amazing afterwards. Even if my hands are cold, my mind feels like it is performing at a better rate.

Cycling

The great thing about cycling is that it provides a cardio workout while working your muscles, whilst being low impact and easier on the knees and ankles than running. Consider investing in an exercise bike. My personal go-to bike is a Peloton, which has changed my morning routine and fitness levels. At first I could not justify the bike in my head financially, but the benefits very quickly became apparent. I can assure you, these bikes will make a world of difference to your life. If it means a few less pairs of Jimmy Choo's, and fewer designer handbags a year, then so be it! The aerobic benefits are the same as with a real bike, and you can cycle in any weather! Use a real bike for leisurely weekend rides. When the weather is fine, I try to cycle to my salon in Westbourne, which is only three miles away. What a difference when I arrive!

Paddleboarding

Fortunately, living by the coast as I do, I have lots of opportunities to paddleboard. I find this so soothing—just me, the paddle, the board, and the water. Bliss. It might surprise you to learn that this uses nearly every muscle group, even during leisurely trips. It requires strength, balance, core muscles, and endurance, yet you wouldn't be able to tell because it's such a fun, relaxing sport.

Aerobic Classes

Aerobic classes can be either low or high impact. Start with low impact, when one foot always stays on the ground, and progress gradually to high impact if you wish. Aerobic classes can have the added benefit of creating a community. When you exercise with others, it helps keep you motivated and on track. There are countless classes, including step, spin, boxing, pilates, yoga, barre, and more. Try them and find out what works for you.

Dancing

Watch or take part in classes in your area, until you find a dance style that appeals to you and that you enjoy. All forms are sociable and fun. Who knows, you might meet Mr/Mrs Right! Dancing provides all the benefits of any regular exercise, but also has the added bonus of extra flexibility and strength.

Variety

My final tip on exercise is to look for variety. If you are just starting out, try out as many different types of exercise as you can. You never know what you might enjoy! Don't get stuck in a single type of exercise or you may find yourself getting bored. Keep it interesting!

Curing Fear of the Gym

If you've never exercised before, or if you have taken a long hiatus, it isn't unusual to feel some anxiety around working out or going to the gym. Some people feel that the gym is only for fit people, while others feel that they will be judged if they look like they don't know what they're doing. It's important not to let these kinds of thoughts interfere with your own goals. Don't let yourself fall into the excuse cycle or get caught up in the expectations of others. Remember, you are doing this for yourself, not to impress others or meet some unspoken expectation of what your fitness regime should look like.

Keep your intention and goals in mind when you are embarking on exercise or going to the gym. Start exercising wherever you feel most comfortable. If that is in your living room in front of an exercise video, there's nothing wrong with that. From there, start branching out. If you are going to the gym, make sure you have a plan. What class are you taking? What machines will you use? Having a plan can help you feel more confident.

Any time you try something new, it can hold a certain element of anxiety around the unknown. Don't let that be a reason not to get healthy.

The Other Side of Exercise

Hopefully, we are now all on the same page when it comes to the importance of exercise. But I can't leave the "Well Be Me" chapter without talking about the other important factor in wellness—meditation! Finding time in your day for stillness is just as important as finding time in the day to be active. And no, sitting in front of your computer for five hours straight doesn't count as stillness! I have already mentioned the importance of your mental health when it comes to committing to a clean lifestyle. A big part of that is meditation.

Of course, if you're having reservations, I get it! If you have never meditated before, you may be saying to yourself, 'How on earth could sitting silently for a few minutes a day have any impact on my health at all?' You aren't alone in this kind of judgement, but meditation has studied and proven benefits. Meditation can reduce stress and anxiety in both the short and long term. Regular meditation practise has also been shown to reduce depression, improve mental health, increase self-awareness, and improve age-related memory loss. In studies, participants who practised meditation were found to report an overall better mental health and quality of life. Studies point to the overwhelming support and improvement of mental capacity and functioning through meditation. Older participants with normal age-related memory loss were found to have improved mental quickness, increased attention span, and a higher ability to complete memory tasks. Even patients with dementia saw improvement in their cognitive functioning after consistent meditation practice.

Aside from markedly improving your mental health, meditation can also improve your physical body. Regular meditation practise has been shown to reduce high blood pressure, improve sleep, reduce insomnia, reduce pain, and some studies even point to an improvement with irritable bowel syndrome. When you meditate, you are opening up and activating different areas of the brain, which in turn alters the way your mind and body react. While that may sound like mumbo jumbo, science has backed up this claim. Studies have found that mindful meditation helps to control pain, without using the naturally occurring opiates. In other words, when you are meditating, your brain is finding new ways to function better.

The mind-body connection is real, so don't dismiss it simply because it's outside of your comfort zone or something you have never done before. We live in a world filled with overstimulation, nearly constant stress, and heightened expectations on our time and performance. It's no wonder that finding mindful stillness has such a profound impact on our wellbeing, because there is no longer space in our lives to allow for it. So, to get those benefits, we need to consciously make time and space to rest.

My Meditation Routine

Over time, you will find your own meditation routine. Until then, you can follow what I do. It lasts only for the count of twelve breaths, or about two minutes. That means it's something you can fit in just about anywhere:

- First, lie down on the floor with your knees bent and the soles of your feet flat on the floor. Knock your knees towards each other so they are lightly touching. Close your eyes, as this immediately helps to calm your central nervous system.

- Scan your body, beginning with your feet. Move up to the ankles, lower legs, knees, upper legs, hips, abdomen, waist, chest, lower back, middle back, upper back, shoulders, throat, jaw, cheeks, eye sockets, eyebrows, forehead, back of the head, and top of the head. As you scan your body, remind each individual part of you to relax. Often, we don't even recognise that we walk through the day with tensed muscles.

- Once you have finished the body scan, bring your focus to your breath. Make each inhale and exhale slow and purposeful. Even if you are brand new to meditation, you should notice a change in your body and a relaxation of the mind relatively quickly.

- Silently repeat the inhale. Now, breathe in, exhale, then breathe out for twelve long, slow breaths.

If you are ready for more or want some variety, check out my favourite apps—CALM and Daily Yoga. There are countless meditation and mindfulness apps out there, but these are the two that I have had good experiences with. CALM is a paid app that provides a new meditation each day, including guided sleep and relaxation. Daily Yoga is a free app that provides at-home yoga routines, along with guided meditation and deep breathing exercises.

Bringing It All Together

I am sure this chapter didn't come as much of a surprise. There is no avoiding the message coming from all directions that we need exercise to be healthy. You should be starting to recognise that everything in your body and everything you do to or with your body works together. Your body is its own system, that reacts to all the forces at play. It's like driving on the highway; all the cars move along efficiently until that one person stops short, causing traffic jams for miles. The same is true for your body. Any one element in misalignment results in a chain of negative consequences.

But, the connection between exercise and skin, hair and nail health, is even more direct than simply keeping your system functioning smoothly. The sweat you produce during exercise flushes out the toxins that are hanging out in your skin. These same toxins can block the pores around your hair follicles. Remember that stress causes your body to overproduce the hormone cortisone, which can cause hair follicles to stop growing. That means the proven stress-reducing effects of exercise and meditation can limit cortisone production, and get your locks growing again!

Try This

The goal of this chapter is simply to get you moving. Whether you are in the habit of exercise or have never had a regular routine, it is time to get committed. Make a plan and stick to it.

First, make a commitment to how much exercise you will get this week. This commitment statement will be different for everyone.

This week I commit to:_____

_____

_____

Next, make a schedule. A commitment statement by itself isn't enough. You need an actionable plan to keep you accountable. Be realistic about your prior commitments, your energy levels, and your interests. Your end goal after a few weeks of acclimatisation should be to get at least twenty minutes of exercise a day. I cannot stress enough that this doesn't have to be formal exercise or even strenuous work. Anything to get you up and moving. On busy days, try to find ways to get moving in your house.

Here is an example of a quick and easy, no-equipment workout, that you can practise on busier days.

Spell your name & do the workout!			
A:	15 push ups	N:	10 push ups
B:	50 jumping jacks	O:	20 lunges
C:	20 crunches	P:	10 tricep dips
D:	10 purpees	Q:	20 jumping jacks
E:	60-second wall sit	R:	60-second plank
F:	20 arm circles	S:	30 bicycle crunches
G:	20 squats	T:	60-second wall sit
H:	30 jumping jacks	U:	40 knee highs
I:	60-second plank	V:	30 squats
J:	20 mountain climbers	W:	15 tricep dips
K:	40 crunches	X:	10 mountain climbers
L:	12 burpees	Y:	12 jumping lunges
M:	15 squat jumps	Z:	30 crunches

No need for a gym or expensive equipment. Repeat this workout three times. If you're feeling strong, repeat it five times. If you get bored of doing your own name, then mix it up! Choose your favourite actress or actor's name, your children's names, or your partner's name. After completing this once, rest for thirty seconds, and then repeat.

Healthy Hair, Happy Body

Fill out the daily chart. Make sure you include what workout you will do and what time of day you will do it.

Sunday	Workout	
Saturday	Workout	
Friday	Workout	
Thursday	Workout	
Wednesday	Workout	
Tuesday	Workout	
Monday	Workout	

Chapter Eight: SLEEP EASY

It isn't hard to recognise the signs of a poor night's sleep: dark circles under your eyes, grogginess, short temper. We all know that we need more sleep, but the deeper side effects that happen under the surface are less well known. At night, while you are sleeping, your body is actually hard at work.

During sleep, your body is in an anabolic state, which means that rather than breaking down the molecules of your body as it does in a catabolic state, it is actually *rebuilding* your body. A catabolic state is often referred to when talking about exercise, because when you exercise you are forcing your body to break down muscle tissue faster. In the anabolic state, your body is growing and repairing. This type of repair and growth is vital for your body's wellbeing. If you spend time at the gym getting exercise, but then don't get a good night's sleep, you are actually making it harder for your body to build muscles or improve your fitness.

But, the work your body does in the anabolic state is so much more than just building your muscles. When in an anabolic state, your body resets your immune system, hormone regulation, nervous system, cardiac system, and organs. This means that without sleep, you are more likely to get sick, have high blood pressure, or migraines. You can even increase your risk of diabetes because of the link to your metabolism. That metabolism link can also leave you feeling hungrier following a poor night's sleep. Sleep helps control your appetite by suppressing hunger hormones and producing leptin, known for regulating appetite.

Healthy Hair, Happy Body

Sleep is important for your brain too. Your brain needs sleep to maintain brain plasticity, which is a fancy way of describing your brain's ability to accept new input. If you don't get enough sleep, you'll have a harder time processing what you have learned during the day, and have a harder time remembering it in the future.

Some studies have found that sleep also encourages the removal of wastes from the brain. This might sound surprising to you, but just like every other organ, our brains do produce waste. However, unlike the other organs, it isn't such a simple job to remove said wastes. Our bodies are constantly moving fluid along the blood vessels of the brain in order to flush the toxins out. Build-up of waste in the brain has been linked to Alzheimer's, amongst other things, and the same studies have shown that getting adequate sleep is vital to this important system. Lack of sleep has also been linked to the onset of neurodegeneration, due in large part to poor waste removal.

So you see, missing that essential sleep can be as detrimental to your health as eating junk food or being sedentary. A poor night's sleep can lead to mood changes, poor concentration, and lack of alertness. When we have many nights of subpar sleep, it can lead to even more serious consequences like heart disease, diabetes, infection, illness, and stroke.

Studies show that one third of Britons sleep for only five or six hours a night, with 27% reporting poor or inadequate sleep regularly. It is still the widely held belief amongst doctors and scientists who study sleep, that eight hours a night is the optimal amount of time. Imagine all of the lurking, unresolved health problems that might be cured simply by getting more sleep.

What Is Getting in the Way?

So, if we should be sleeping way more than we are, what exactly is preventing so many of us from getting our much-needed sleep? The answer, of course, is different for everyone. However, there are a few areas of concern that most commonly interfere with sleep.

One of our biggest problems goes back to biology. Humans are naturally diurnal, which means we are awake during the day and asleep at night. Our biology has developed to support this habit with our circadian rhythm. Our circadian rhythm tells us when to start feeling tired and when to wake up. The problem is, we've learned how to trick our circadian rhythm. Our brains (and our circadian rhythm) interpret artificial light in the same way as natural sunlight, so staring at our screens well after the sun has gone down tricks our body into thinking it isn't yet time for sleep. We also throw off our system by simply not listening to our circadian rhythm. The demands of regular life—work, kids, and household chores—all mean that even when we are feeling tired and ready for sleep, we can't simply climb into bed. Instead, we stay awake, pushing our bodies past when they should naturally be asleep.

Artificial light and responsibility aren't the only things keeping us from catching the right amount of sleep. Stress, diet, and sedentary lifestyles all play a part in us having trouble sleeping. According to The Telegraph newspaper, almost half (44%) of all Britons report dealing with some form of stress. The problem with stress is that it both causes and is caused by poor sleep, creating a terrible cycle which is hard to break. The same chemicals connected with deep sleep also tell the body to stop producing stress hormones. That means that if you aren't reaching deep sleep, you also aren't turning off the stress hormones either. The opposite is also true. When you're stressed, it's harder to sleep. Stress hormones peak in late afternoon and evening, which means as you are starting to settle in for the night, your stress is ramping up.

Your diet can affect your sleep in some surprising ways too. It isn't just what you eat that leaves you tossing and turning. Eating too much or too little can have a real impact on your quality of sleep. Eating too late can also cause problems.If you are eating large meals too close to bedtime, you are setting yourself up for disrupted sleep. What you eat, of course, is also important. Eating sugary, processed foods, foods with hidden MSGs, or loading up on caffeine throughout the day, will leave you jittery, sluggish, and unable to sleep.

Studies by the National Sleep Foundation found that a sedentary lifestyle is a direct factor in poor sleep. Exercise is known to decrease stress and anxiety (as we talked about in the last chapter) and can physically exhaust your body, making it easier to sleep. Without any sort of physical activity, you are more likely to be sitting down for most of the day, staring at a screen and often overstimulating your brain. It is no wonder that being sedentary leads to sleep issues!

Getting Help

There are two ways to get help, the right way and the wrong way. Too often, people are looking for a quick fix in the same way they are looking for a quick fix for losing weight or getting healthy. If you have been paying attention so far, you'll probably understand that the *right way* to improve your sleep involves working hard, getting healthy, and being honest with yourself about your current unhealthy habits. The *wrong way* is relying on synthetic quick fixes that in the end only make things worse.

Sleep Aids to Avoid

One in ten people have consulted their doctor about sleep, but three times as many have taken medication to help their sleep. That means that far too many people are self-medicating when it comes to sleep.

It can be really tempting to take a "magic" pill to knock you out at night and solve all of your problems. But sleeping pills come with a high price tag, and don't always guarantee better sleep. When you take a sleeping pill, you are inducing an artificial sleep by releasing chemicals that bind onto your neurotransmitters, causing them to slow down transmissions. This means that, despite being able to fall asleep, you may not wake up feeling very rested at all.

All sleeping medicines have side-effects, but before we start getting into that, let's talk about the drawbacks of sleeping pills themselves. It is common that once you start taking sleeping pills, you can develop a drug tolerance. As you take the medicine more consistently over time, it will become less and less effective. That means that you need to up your dosage to get the same effect, which of course increases the likelihood and severity of side-effects. Sleeping pills are also known to be very addictive, leaving you with worse insomnia and withdrawal symptoms if you skip a dose or stop taking them. Sleeping pills can also interact in dangerous ways with other medications and drugs. At this point you have to ask yourself, is it worth it? You are not solving your problem, instead you are masking it and putting it off for another day. Unless you plan on taking sleeping pills your entire life—DON'T! You are simply prolonging the problem and making it worse in the process.

The side effects of sleeping pills range from the mildly annoying, like dry mouth, next-day drowsiness (again, what's the point in taking a sleeping pill just to feel sluggish and drowsy the next day?), constipation, and lack of balance, to the truly dangerous. The latter includes issues like memory loss, hallucinations, suicidal thoughts, sleepwalking, and sleep-driving (yes, that is a thing!). We have become desensitised to side effects in this age of over-prescribed medicine, but none of these are worth brushing aside. Any one of these alone outweighs any benefits you might gain from a sleep aid. Sleep is important, but getting synthetic, drug-induced sleep is counter-productive to your goal of getting healthy!

Alcohol

Alcohol may reduce the amount of time it takes to fall asleep, but it can also significantly increase sleep disturbance. Drinking before bed has been known to cause more abrupt transitions between your sleep stages. That can lead to more frequent wake-ups and nightmares. Alcohol can also cause increased snoring and in some cases sleep apnoea. It affects your core body temperature, making it harder to stay comfortable, and induces night sweats.

We are all, probably, adults here and if you want to have an occasional drink or even more than an occasional drink, that is your decision to make.

My suggestions for alcohol include:

- Have regular alcohol-free days.

- Don't drink for two consecutive days.

- Choose the purest alcohol you can.

- If it's wine, opt for a less sugary option such as Sauvignon Blanc, Pinot Grigio, Merlot, or Pinot Noir.

- The best choice you can make is grain-free vodka with soda.

- Mix alcohol with soda, tonic, or water. Never use mixers.

- Choose red wine over white.

- Drink water before and after to avoid dehydration.

- Choose organic wines.

- Remember that if your liver is too busy trying to remove alcohol from your body, some of its energy for handling ageing hormones will be diverted!

Healthy Ways to Improve Your Sleep

Don't get discouraged by the dangers and ineffectiveness of medicines to aid sleep. Better sleep is possible! And it is within YOUR power.

Exercise for Sleep

As we discussed earlier, not getting exercise makes quality sleep harder to come by. But, the good news is that getting exercise, even if it is light aerobic exercise, can drastically improve your sleep. People who exercise five to six times a week are the least likely to take sleep medication or consult a doctor with regards to sleep-related issues.

Diet

Once again, what you eat affects how well your body functions, and that includes how well you sleep. If you follow my clean eating guide, you should start seeing an improvement in sleep. That's because you will have cut out sugar, limited caffeine, and increased healthy fats, proteins, fruits, and vegetables. It isn't a surprise that caffeine and sugar will wreak havoc on your sleep. Both are stimulants and cause inflammation in your gut. Your goal is to get your body back in balance, so it can do its job!

Getting Out in the Sun

We talked about your circadian rhythm getting out of whack from too much artificial light. The best way to remedy this is to get out in the natural sunlight. The sunlight will help reset your natural, internal body clock. It also provides you with vitamin D. Low levels of vitamin D have been linked to poor and restless sleep. According to one study, half the world's population is suffering from vitamin D deficiency. Another study saw a marked improvement in sleep and neurological problems when the subjects raised their vitamin D levels.

Establishing a Routine

A quick Google search of how to improve sleep will pull up loads of articles referencing the importance of a bedtime routine. I know what you're thinking: you gave up a bedtime routine at seven years old when your parents stopped reading you a story and tucking you in. Yet, it is unrealistic to assume that your mind can go from one hundred to zero in a minute, so you need to prepare for it.

Leading up to bedtime, you need to send your mind and body warning signals that it is time to start unwinding. Unlike some of the other techniques for better sleep, a bedtime routine isn't something that happens because of the chemicals in your body or what you are or aren't eating. Instead, it is simply about retraining yourself to create a calming environment, leading up to when you rest your head on your pillow.

The power of habit is very strong. In his book *The Power of Habit,* Charles Duhigg references the "habit loop" in which we get a cue that leads us to perform an action, which provides some type of reward. For example, you may start exercising because you just read this book and you want to start getting healthier. That is your initial cue, so you go out and work up a good sweat, but exercise becomes a habit *because* you start seeking that endorphin reward.

Habits can go both ways. Sometimes we form bad habits, like scrolling through our Facebook newsfeed right before bed to see what all our friends did that day. Other times, the habits we form help us, like brushing our teeth every day. You have a bedtime routine, even if you don't know it. The goal is to make your habits work better for you. When I said the power of better sleep is in YOUR hands, I meant it! This is the most effective thing you can do for yourself.

Falling into Routine

The big question now, is how do we create a bedtime routine, and what should it look like? Well, the first step is making sure you have enough time to both sleep and go through a routine. Your aim should be seven to eight hours a night of shut-eye. I always start preparing for bed a good hour before I intend to sleep.

Your bedtime routine can consist of whatever is most helpful and practical to you, but here are some things to consider.

During the Day:

- Spend some time during the day moving your body and working up a sweat.

- Try to stop eating around 7:00 p.m., to give your body time to finish digesting before you lie down for bed. You don't want your body working when it should be resting.

- Don't nap during the day. If you can't help yourself, at least don't do it after 3:00 p.m.

- If you choose to drink coffee throughout the day, you must be blessed with the gene that breaks down caffeine particularly fast. Otherwise, don't drink coffee after lunch.

- No watching TV or looking at your phone in bed. Your bed should be for sleeping in (and sex), nothing else.

- Say goodbye to weekend lie-ins. Set your alarm clock to wake up at the same time every morning. This creates a ritual, and you know how much your body loves a ritual!

Getting Ready for Bed:

- Be in bed by 10:30 p.m. at least four nights a week. That means you should start your routine around 9:30 p.m.

- Turn off your phone and the TV one hour before bed. Instead, try something more relaxing like meditation or a hot bath.

- Before you go to sleep, write down three good things that happened to you that day.

- Having a warm bath or hot shower at least an hour before bed can also be helpful, but be sure to cool down before you go to bed, as this temperature drop tells your brain that it's time to sleep. (See my recipe for a lavender bath in the next section.)

- Sleep in a cool room; I always sleep with my window open.

- A snack, such as an oatmeal biscuit or a banana, may help you get to sleep. Or, try a fabulous peanut and banana smoothie.

- Many herbal teas claim to ensure a good night's sleep. Chamomile, lime blossom, and valerian are said to be the most effective. Stir a spoonful of honey into your chamomile tea, as it's known for its sedative properties.

- Invest in an aromatherapy diffuser. My favourite brand has been Tisserand Aroma Spa. I use it to diffuse essential oils that encourage and aid sleep. For myself, I use lavender, and for my children I use Roman chamomile.

- If sex is on the menu, there's nothing better than a rip-roaring orgasm to release every angst in the body. But, if it isn't, and you haven't got a sex toy in your bedside cabinet, you need to educate your body and mind that it's time for sleep. You can do this by establishing a proper bedtime routine.

- If all this fails, don't lie awake for hours worrying; get up and do something useful but relaxing for twenty minutes or so, until you feel tired.

> Your body loves a ritual!

Lavender Bath

Lavender immediately fills me with a sense of calm, so much so that I spray my pillow with lavender oil at bedtime. I've found that after a particularly hideous day, this simple act can dramatically alter my mood and promote a good night's sleep. One of my favourite ways to relax is to take a Lavender/Epsom salt bath.

The following blend is especially suited to ease tired aches and pains. I always add more Epsom salts than the recipe suggests, as this makes it feel far more therapeutic:

3 cups = 1 bath

You will need:

1 cup sea salt

2 cups Epsom salts

20 drops lavender essential oil

Mix all the ingredients together in a large bowl. Use immediately or store the salts in an airtight glass container for later use.

To use, add the entire batch to a bath of warm water, and soak as long as desired. Take a quick shower afterwards to rinse off the salts.

Bringing It All Together

Alright, if everything I have said so far about sleep hasn't convinced you to get your sleep habits in order, this should get you going. Just one night of bad sleep can make adults age faster! That means that all the hard work you are doing to eat healthily, drink your water, exercise, and meditate is being undone when you aren't getting the shut-eye you need. The American Academy of Sleep Medicine found that lack of sleep directly impacts the process of biological ageing. The study looked at the impact of poor sleep on gene patterns, and found that the patterns were consistent with faster ageing. This applies to your skin, hair, and nails just as much as everything else. Another study found that participants who didn't get enough sleep showed signs of fine lines, uneven pigmentation, and reduced skin elasticity!

Beyond triggering the ageing systems of the body, lack of sleep also breaks down your skin's natural functions. At night, when you are sleeping, your body sends out hormones which stimulate the production of skin cells and collagen. Naturally, these contribute to healthier hair and skin. If you're not sleeping, the body instead releases the harmful cortisol-stress hormone that we have already talked about. This leads to inflammation. The lack of collagen leads to lines, wrinkles, and an increase in acne. In fact, a study by the British Medical Journal found that people who had a full night's sleep were healthier, less tired, and deemed more attractive by outside observers than those who didn't get enough sleep. The saying about getting your beauty sleep wasn't wrong! If you don't like those fine lines and wrinkles, then don't skimp on your sleep!

Try This

It's time to create your own personalised bedtime routine. As you start thinking about your routine, keep your own personal preferences and daily limitations in mind. You don't want your routine to eat up too much of your day, be too short, or be too unrealistic. That being said, there are some things that I am going to *insist* be part of your routine.

My bedtime will be:

Monday	Tuesday	Wednesday	Thursday	Friday	Saturday	Sunday

During the day I will:

Come up with three things you will do differently during the day to improve your sleep. Suggestions include cutting out coffee, increasing exercise, removing a nap, setting an alarm in the morning, not working from bed, etc.

1. _____

   _____

2. _____

   _____

3. _____

   _____

One hour before bed I will:

List four things that you will do in the hour before bed tonight. This list can be modified as you figure out what works and what doesn't work for you, but we are going to stick to it for a full week.

1. Turn off my phone an hour before bed.

2. _____

    _____

3. _____

    _____

4. _____

    _____

Reflection

Whatever modifications you choose to add or remove from your day and night, I want you to continue them for a full week before making any changes to your routine. A bedtime routine isn't magic. It isn't going to make you Sleeping Beauty in a single night. It takes time to see what is working. Each morning for a full week, I want you to come back to this page and reflect upon your sleep the previous night, by answering a couple of questions. When the week is over, you can tweak your routine and continue, until you feel that your routine is the best it can be.

Day One	Answer	Notes
Did you do everything on your list?		
Did you get in bed on time?		
How long did it take you to fall asleep?		
Did you sleep through the night? If not, how many times did you wake?		
How rested did you feel in the morning?		

Chapter Nine: KEEPING MY LOCKS

If you have ever been on Facebook and browsed the internet, you have probably seen advertisements for miracle hair growth shampoos or secret elixirs that are guaranteed to make your hair grow by inches and become fuller overnight. Hopefully, by this point in the book, you are starting to realise that hair growth doesn't really start at the scalp. Using fancy shampoos and rubbing oils on your head isn't going to do much if you aren't solving the problem that is *causing* the poor growth.

How Does Hair Grow, Anyway?

Although it may seem strange, you can think of your hair like a plant. The follicle at the base of your hair is like a seed, and from that seed your hair grows. At the bottom of each "seed" or follicle, the roots spread out. These roots are made up of protein cells. The roots pull nutrients and hormones from the blood and send them to the follicle, making your hair grow. The nutrients provide the materials to make up the hair, while the hormones tell the hair when to grow.

Each follicle spends about three to five years in the growing phase, called the anagen phase. Then it transitions into the catagen phase, in which the hair detaches from the blood supply and stops growing for about three weeks. The last phase, telogen, is when your hair prepares to shed and eventually falls out, taking about three months before the cycle starts over again.

Healthy Hair, Happy Body

Luckily, different strands of hair are at different stages at different times, so we don't go temporarily bald every few years! About 80% of your hair follicles are in the anagen phase at the same time. It is normal for healthy adults to shed between 50-100 hairs each day because new hairs are developing. Researchers believe that the anagen phase is mostly predetermined by your genetics. That means if you are predisposed to a shorter anagen phase, your hair will probably not grow very long.

A lot of what your hair looks like, feels like, and grows like may be genetic, but—and that is a big but—anything that interrupts this natural cycle can change the length of your anagen phase! It is a fragile ecosystem that needs to be in perfect balance to function the way it's supposed to. If your hormones are off, they may be telling your hair follicles to cut the anagen phase short, making your hair fall out more often. If you aren't getting the proper nutrition, then your hair isn't going to grow properly. Your hair is a non-vital system, so if your diet is poor then those important nutrients are being redirected to your more vital systems.

Unfortunately, it is easier for your hair to be out of balance and unhealthy than it is for it to be healthy and balanced, especially if you aren't taking the time and making the effort. Anything from overly restricted calories, to childbirth, to major life changes, can impact how your hair grows. If you add to that any underlying health problems, like circulatory problems, thyroid disorders, irritable bowel syndrome or endometritis as I experienced, you may face serious hair loss. It is no surprise then that eight million women in the UK suffer from hair loss, and 40% of men will experience notable hair loss by the age of 35.

Hair loss can be more devastating than people imagine. It carries with it a social stigma, health worries, and of course self-esteem troubles. When I suffered hair loss in my teens and late twenties, my self-esteem was ravaged. I worked in a high-powered job, and imagined that everyone was judging me based on my hair health.

Common Reasons for Hair Loss

We have talked a lot throughout this book about how you can start to improve your health by taking small steps right away. If you've followed all of the advice up until this point, you should start seeing some improvements, but it is important to understand what type of hair loss you may have. This will help you work toward specific improvements.

Male Pattern Hair Loss

Simply put, male pattern hair loss is usually inherited from the maternal grandfather (love you too, Grandad!). It starts either with a recession to the temples or a diffuse thinning to the crown, and is generally followed by a gradual thinning, then a total loss of hair on the top of your head. It's rare that hair loss occurs at the side and back.

With male pattern baldness, the hair isn't actually gone. People living without male pattern baldness presumably have infinite cycles of hair growth, shedding and regrowth, yet men who inherited the baldness gene continue to cycle through. With each regrowth, their hair becomes thinner and thinner, until it is nearly non-existent.

Female Pattern Hair Loss

Unlike male pattern baldness, female pattern hair loss doesn't have a single, easy to identify cause. Instead, it can be caused by a few different reasons. The first is still genetic. Some women are simply genetically predisposed to lose their hair in the same way men do. Another leading reason is hormonal fluctuations. Discontinuing birth control, getting pregnant, or any of the other many hormonal changes that women go through in any given month can lead to increased hair loss. Some women are more sensitive to increased testosterone levels, which can then wreak havoc on your hair.

Female pattern hair loss presents as a thinning to the front and crown area of the scalp, similar to male pattern baldness. Again, balding never occurs at the sides and back. Your hair parting can appear wider, and the scalp can seem more noticeable at the front and the top of the head if you suffer from female pattern hair loss.

Telogen Effluvium (Symptomatic/Reflective Loss)

If you are noticing a large number of hairs in your brush or comb, particularly when you've just washed your hair, you may be experiencing the most common type of excess hair shedding—acute telogen effluvium (ATE), or its prolonged counterpart, chronic telogen effluvium (CTE). On examination of the scalp, many hairs will come away with only minor traction. You may also notice many short, re-growing, tapered hairs of similar length through the scalp with ATE, whereas with CTE your hair will shed relentlessly, resulting in a loss of hair density and an apparent thinning at partings. With CTE, regrowth is still present but at differing lengths.

Unfortunately, there isn't nearly enough research on any of the telogen effluvium conditions to fully understand why it starts or why it stops. ATE is essentially when you have fewer hair follicles growing hair. That means that if a number of hair follicles stop producing hair during the telogen phase, the number of dormant hairs increases, leaving you with excessive shedding.

Alopecia Areata

Alopecia areata is an autoimmune disease, which means your immune system starts attacking your own body. In the case of alopecia areata, your immune system attacks your hair follicle. The hair loss that results can vary widely from patient to patient, but can be quite a drastic type of hair loss.

Alopecia areata presents a number of circular completely bald patches, which sometimes merge with other patches and therefore make the hair follicles clearly visible. The earliest patch will often re-grow, but only with fine, white hairs from the centre of the patch. This condition is unpredictable and can last from six months to many years depending on the cause. The condition can cover the whole scalp (alopecia totalis) or the whole body can be affected (alopecia universalis).

Ophiasic Areata

Ophiasic areata is a milder yet more persistent form of alopecia areata and affects the nape area, where the back of the head meets the neck, as well as the front and sides of the scalp.

Traction Alopecia

Most commonly seen in people with hair extensions, or anyone who frequently wears their hair up in a tight style daily, as well as people with hair braids or fitted heavy hair systems, traction alopecia appears on the margins of the scalp and sometimes shows irregular patchy hair loss to the crown area. This is generally caused by excessive chemical or physical trauma through continuous hair styling methods.

Traumatic Hair Loss or Breakage

Trichotillomania is a form of self-inflicted physical trauma and is when one pulls out their own hair through a recognised obsessive-compulsive disorder. Although very common with young children, they often outgrow the habit. This is a far more difficult habit to break in adults.

Scarring Alopecia

Scarring alopecia presents itself as an irregular area of shiny bald skin, which can be a darker or lighter colour than the skin surrounding it. No hair follicles are present, and the skin can be raised. Essentially, when the hair starts to fall out, a scar is formed, making it difficult or impossible to grow a new follicle. Therefore, it does not support normal hair growth. There are three main causes of scarring: chemical, infection, and autoimmune disease.

Other Hair Loss Problems

The majority of patients that come into my salons and clinics suffer from the medical issues that I have just mentioned. But, there are some that come in with less common issues. They suffer from moderate to severe scalp issues that first seem to affect the skin of the scalp before causing hair loss.

Eczema

Those suffering from eczema can be dismayed when it breaks out on their scalp, as it is so difficult to contain and heal. Eczema is a blanket term for a number of different skin conditions that all present similarly. It is characterised by excessively dry, itchy skin that can appear scaly, red, and raised. When eczema is on the scalp, it can also result in hair loss. A number of different causes can attribute to eczema, including genetics, hormones, autoimmune diseases, other skin conditions, and even depression.

Dermatitis

Sometimes eczema can be confused with dermatitis—this occurs when concentrations of shampoos, conditioners, or other hair products are applied to the scalp and cause inflammation as opposed to an allergic reaction.

Far more severe, is allergic dermatitis. Apart from being potentially life-threatening, this irritable reaction happens when a substance previously applied on the skin is re-applied. A reaction can happen hours or days after application, but can spread to the eyes and face, causing infection. At worst, there can be an anaphylactic shock, causing restriction of the windpipe.

Psoriasis

Often beginning on the elbows, knees, and shins, psoriasis is dry and white with silvery scales lined with bleeding points that can be seen underneath them. No one has really gotten to the root of the problem, but it is definitely triggered by stress. A more critical form is pityriasis amiantacea, which weeps. It is especially difficult to live with when the main symptom is prolonged intense inching.

Acne Necrotica

Acne necrotica miliaris is when the hair follicles "open", causing tiny scars when they heal, which leads to hair loss.

Ringworm

Ringworm doesn't actually involve any type of worms, but it is a fungal infection of the scalp. It causes non-scarring patchy hair loss, showing brittle hairs and broken stumps of hair, which are grey-coloured regardless of the colour of the surrounding hair.

HELP!

As I mentioned before, it's important to ignore the nearly endless pop-up ads, all of them trying to convince you that the hair product they are touting is the single miracle product you need. It's a lie! I am not saying every product out there doesn't work, simply that all of those products can't possibly work for everyone. Let me explain. There isn't one single cause of hair loss, therefore there will never be one single fix. Those serums, tonics, shampoos, and oils may be the right fix for some causes of hair loss, but not for every cause. More often than not, they only work for one type of hair loss.

While all of the things we have talked about so far in this book—a healthy gut, clean living, limiting sugar, cupboard love, drinking water, exercising, and getting sleep—are absolutely essential to your health and therefore healthy hair, you still have to understand your hair loss in order to best address it. To be absolutely clear, you cannot expect to skip over all the other steps in this book, come to this chapter, and only follow the advice in this section to then start growing the best hair of your life. Everything you do to and for your body has a ripple effect. Everything either encourages health or discourages it. You cannot expect to take a supplement like Simone Thomas Wellness, while eating McDonald's every night, and be healthy or have nice hair.

That being said, the reverse is true too. Lustrous hair that looks and feels fantastic requires a whole spectrum of healthy beauty nutrients to keep it well-conditioned, healthy, and strong. If you want to improve your hair health, getting healthy is step one. Step two is guaranteeing you have the right nutrients for your hair. It took me many years to discover the key nutrients that specifically feed and nourish my own hair.

So now, let's look at some of these key nutrients. Some of these will overlap with the nutrients that I listed in the "Clean Living" chapter. Your body and mind need a wide variety of nutrients to function at peak performance, but not all of them directly affect the hair. In order to help my clients navigate the complex and often confusing world of nutrients and supplements, I have made a line of supplements specifically designed for hair health, gut health, and anti-aging, plus helping with detoxification. At the time of writing, I have won The Independent newspaper's "Best Buy Indy" award. The Independent tested a range of hair supplements, and the Simone Thomas Wellness Hair Care Plans came number 1 for best-tasting, most effective supplements! Participants tested both the Biotin and the Ginkgo Hair Care Plans and were "astounded by the results". Testers also highlighted that results were consistent and noticeable within four weeks, and were impressed by the vegan-friendly, completely natural and easy-to-swallow capsules in each plan. Again, that doesn't mean you need to buy from me if you would prefer finding your own. But, I genuinely believe I can offer you the best treatment available. So, give it a go!

Iron

If there are low levels of iron in the body, then this can often lead to mild or severe hair loss. When our diets are lacking in iron, the scalp may not receive adequate nutrients and oxygen. Thus, hair becomes dull, brittle, and fragile. With this in mind, it's essential to include good sources of iron in your daily diet.

FEED ME: Leafy Greens, Nuts, Oats, Seeds, Fish, Wholegrains, Pulses and Figs.

Water

We have talked about water before, but I cannot underestimate the importance of drinking enough. Water assists in efficient and healthy hair growth, making almost a quarter of the weight of a hair strand. I drink two litres of water every day, in order to get gleaming and healthy tresses. Remember that filtered water is best, or water from a glass bottle—avoid drinking water from a plastic bottle!

Antioxidants

These protective plant compounds help to strengthen the tiny capillaries near the surface of our skin. In turn, this promotes a healthy circulation to the scalp, nourishing the hair shaft while keeping hair glossy and strong.

FEED ME: Berries, Beetroot, Peppers, Squash, Tomatoes.

Vitamin A

Remember, your hair is made up of cells, and all cells need vitamin A in order to grow. Vitamin A also helps us produce an oily substance called sebum. Sebum moisturises the scalp and keeps hair healthy. People with a deficiency in this vitamin may experience dull hair or hair loss.

FEED ME: Eggs, Carrots, Leafy Greens, Sweet Potatoes, Dried Apricots.

Vitamin B

Various studies show that a deficiency in vitamin B (also called biotin) can cause hair loss too. Biotin helps red blood cells to carry nutrients and oxygen to the scalp and hair follicles, both of which are vital for the hair to grow.

FEED ME: Simone Thomas Wellness Biotin or the Ginkgo Hair Care Plan, Eggs, Meat, Leafy Greens, Sunflower Seeds, Almonds, Avocado, Brown Rice.

Vitamin C

Vitamin C is essential for forming collagen—the structural protein that holds the hair together. Hair follicles, blood vessels, and the scalp all need collagen to stay healthy. Even a moderate lack of vitamin C can have a detrimental effect on our hair, leaving it dry, brittle and lacklustre.

FEED ME: Simone Thomas Wellness SkinQuencher, Citrus Fruits, Kiwi, Berries, Broccoli, Kale, Peppers, Sweet Potatoes, Tomato Juice, Eggs.

Calcium

While most people associate calcium with bone health, calcium also helps with the secretion of hormones and enzymes. Even if you're getting lots of vitamin B, you still need calcium; otherwise the biotin enzyme isn't going to make its way to your hair. When it comes to my dairy-free family, we've had to find new sources of calcium.

FEED ME: Anchovies, Pilchards, Whitebait, Broccoli, Bok Choy, Cabbage, Chard, Kale, Rocket, Watercress, Pulses, Chickpeas, Kidney Beans, Lentils, Peanuts, Brown Rice, Quinoa, Nuts, Seeds, Tahini, Fruits, Figs, Rhubarb.

Essential Fatty Acids

These important fats help to balance sebum production in the body, which in turn keeps the scalp healthy and the hair looking glossy and well-conditioned. As our bodies can't make the vital omega-3 and omega-6 required, we need to eat foods that are plentiful in these essential fats.

FEED ME: Chia, Flaxseeds, Hemp, Pumpkin, Sunflower Seeds, Avocado, Nuts, Seaweed, Oily Fish, Simone Thomas Wellness Super Green Supplements.

High-Quality Protein

Protein is the building block for every muscle, cell, and hair on our bodies. It is essential for strong, healthy growth. Insufficient protein can slow hair growth and lead to brittle hair strands.

FEED ME: Nuts, Seeds, Pulses, Fish, Lean Meat.

Sulphur

The beauty mineral sulphur helps to build strong, healthy hair, as it is essential for holding keratin—the main hair protein—in shape. It strengthens hair and aids the absorption of other important proteins.

FEED ME: Cauliflower, Cabbage, Broccoli, Brussels Sprouts, Onion, Garlic.

Zinc

Zinc helps to balance the production of sebum from the sebaceous glands at the base of the hair follicle, which in turn encourages hair growth, promotes a healthy, flake-free scalp, and ensures hair is well-conditioned.

FEED ME: Unrefined Grains, Peaches, Pomegranates, Cashew, Pumpkin Seeds, Sesame Seeds, Lentils.

Silica

Silica is a vital mineral for hair health, as it's essential for the production of collagen. Silica helps the body absorb other vital minerals and vitamins, taking nutrients to the peripheries of the body and ensuring that hair follicles get the nutrients they need.

FEED ME: Cucumber, Oats, Flaxseeds, Avocado, Onions, Mango.

Try This

First and foremost, if you suspect that you have any of the medical problems listed in this book, make an appointment with your doctor right away. Or, alternatively, you can make an appointment with me and my team for a bioenergetic screening. Even if you live outside of the UK, it isn't a problem, because we work with clients all over the world! My clients send me samples including nail clippings, hair, and saliva that I can analyse to help you create a personalised plan. It's never a good idea to use a book to diagnose and treat real medical issues, no matter how amazing that book may be! Instead, make sure you treat this book as a healthy lifestyle guide, which can supplement and support advice from a specialist.

When new clients walk through my doors, rather than sitting them down in a chair and going straight to work on a solution, we spend the time assessing the problem. Within a 90-minute consultation, we look at food, lifestyle, and health history, as well as family history, along with bioenergetic testing and screening. There are countless factors that can affect hair health. Giving my clients a one-size-fits-all solution wouldn't be the answer. The same goes for you. It is so tempting to try throwing money at the problem—buying any product that has halfway decent reviews—but part of the goal of this book is to change your habits, get healthier, and be more mindful about how you're approaching your life.

Bioenergetics

Bioenergetics focuses on the energy flow of your body and how it can affect your overall health. We recognise that DNA, medicine, drug use, illness, stress, and lifestyle choices can cause inflammation, which then reaches your hair and causes hair loss. It is important to think about your body, mind, health, and hair as a single system working together. A rash on your skin probably isn't just a rash on your skin, but a symptom of a larger issue. Likewise, a headache or stomach-ache isn't disconnected from the rest of your body. In order to have a healthy lifestyle, every part of our body must be working in harmony.

Chapter Ten: KEEPING MY LOOKS

You have twenty square feet of skin on your body, and boy, does it have a big job to do! Your skin is in fact your largest organ, although we don't always think of it that way. It's your body's first defence against infection and disease, and protects all of the vital organs, regulates body temperature, and allows us to feel sensations. When we go out into the sun, our skin has the ability to produce vitamin D, which contributes to our mood regulation, anti-ageing, healthy bones, and a sharp mind. The goal of good skincare is twofold. Of course, we all want youthful, radiant skin, but we also need to make sure that our skin is as healthy as possible, so it can continue to protect us.

Taking Care of Your Skin

Too many people don't start thinking about the health of their skin until they start to see visible signs of ageing damage. But, the truth is, the harmful things that affect our skin can make a noticeable difference within just twenty-four hours.

Have you ever spent a night out with friends and ended up enjoying yourself a little too much? The first thing you notice when you wake up the next day is the pounding headache, but the next thing you notice when you look in the mirror, is your puffy face! This is mostly attributed to dehydration and a change in blood circulation when you drink too much alcohol. And, what's worse is that it isn't just alcohol that can leave your skin dry, lacklustre, puffy, or discoloured. Like our hair, the skin will show signs of poor nutrition and unhealthy habits much faster than anything else in your body (think dark circles when you don't sleep enough). More often than not, we still only treat the damage to our skin from the outside (for more on topical skincare, check out chapter eleven). But what's happening on the outside is a more genuine reflection of what is happening on the *inside*.

Let's cut to the chase. Eating processed foods filled with sugar and preservatives is ageing you! No amount of lotions, creams, serums, or tonics are going to save you from what you are putting into your body. Clean eating is the number one most important thing you can do for your skin and your hair, tied with drinking enough water. The food we eat provides important nutrients, but those nutrients also combat free radicals. You may have heard the term "free radicals" before, but let me throw a little science at you. When we take a breath, oxygen comes into our body as single, unpaired electrons. The problem is that electrons like to be paired, so these single electrons travel throughout your body, searching for a partner. When doing this, they break down the cells that make up other parts of our body, damaging them in the process. That's right, oxygen! The air we need to live is also waging a silent war within our bodies. But, luckily, the nutrients that we find in fruit and vegetables help us. They do this by pairing with oxygen, and cleaning up the free radicals. On the other hand, things like alcohol, cigarettes, and even fried food create *more* free radicals.

We have already talked at length about the importance of drinking enough water, but if you need a refresher then go back and read chapter six again. Our body is made up of 50-70% water. And there is only one way to replenish that—water! If you follow my advice in the previous chapters around diet, exercise, water and sleep, you will soon see that your complexion looks dramatically different.

For an extra boost, you may want to start thinking about collagen. Collagen is the most abundant protein we have, making up about one-third of all the proteins in your body. It's a major building block in bones, skin, muscles, tendons, and ligaments. Collagen is the essential glue that holds these things together, and is also what keeps the face full and youthful. I have a multi-award winning collagen product, called SkinQuencher, which contains vitamin C and essential amino acids. So, check it out, if you haven't already: https://simonethomaswellness.com/products/skin-quencher

Your body stops producing collagen after the age of 25. As we grow older, the connective tissue starts to loosen and the elasticity reduces, causing the face to droop. There's no miracle cream that will reverse the signs of ageing; you can only try to slow down the process. Eating a healthy diet, full of skin-benefitting foods, should be the first step, along with exercise and a good skincare routine.

Healthy Hair, Happy Body

Supplementing your collagen does more than just improve your skin. In numerous studies, people who took collagen supplements in addition to undergoing a strength training regime, showed increased muscle mass beyond those who only did strength training. Another example was when a subject suffering from arthritis reported a marked improvement in pain over the seventy-day study.

Where to Find Collagen

Just like we make collagen, animals do too. It is found in high quantities in chicken and pork skin, but your best natural source of collagen comes from bone broth, made by boiling down the bones of chickens and other animals. I know it doesn't sound too appetising, but it makes a great base for soup, with the added bonus of boosting your collagen. My go-to every winter, or when a family member is unwell, is my chicken bone broth. You can find this on NutriHome.

Collagen Supplements

If you don't have the time or stomach for bone broth, collagen supplements are an easy alternative. Collagen supplements come in two forms, pills or powders, and it is up to personal preference which one you want to start taking. There are three main types of collagen found on the market. Type I is for skin, nails, hair, organs, bones, and ligaments. Type II is mainly for collagen, and Type III is for fibrous protein in bone, cartilage, dentin, tendon, and other connective tissues. Needless to say, Type I is ideal for skin, hair, and beauty health.

Another important factor when looking for collagen is how it is prepared. With any supplement, your body can only absorb and use so much at a time. Collagen is a large protein. Therefore, in order to get anything out of it, it must be hydrolysed. This is a process that breaks it down small enough for your body to use. When taking collagen, it is also important to get enough vitamin C; your body can't effectively use the collagen without this. Some collagens come with vitamin C included, but if you are taking another supplement with vitamin C then you don't need to worry.

My final tip about collagen is, when possible, choose marine collagen. Collagen is available from both marine and bovine sources, and both provide benefits, but marine collagen is smaller and easier to absorb—meaning your body can use more of it. Marine sources also have higher antioxidants (to fight those free radicals we talked about). They contain an amino acid called hydroxyproline, which encourages your skin to increase or start producing its own collagen. Simone Thomas Wellness SkinQuencher's marine collagen is from a certified sustainable source, as this is very important to me.

Food Sensitivities

We've all heard of food allergies. But, just because you don't break out in hives or go into anaphylaxis, that doesn't mean that you can eat whatever you want. I am talking about food sensitivities specifically, which wreak havoc on your body, but are often most apparent in how they affect your skin.

The main difference between a food allergy and a food sensitivity is that an allergy can be life-threatening. Most people know if they have life-threatening allergies, and since that is more concerning than whether your skin looks bad, I am not going to spend time on that here. Instead, I want to talk about food sensitivities. Many people don't even know they have sensitivities. However, it has got to the point where I can immediately tell if someone has a sensitivity to (or is consuming too much of) a certain food or drink, just by looking at their face when they walk into my clinic. Time and time again, the same signs show up on the face. Some of my patients are really in tune with their bodies and can spot foods that cause problems quickly, whereas others have no idea that their skin and health woes are a result of what they're eating. Sometimes people live with food sensitivities their whole life, and therefore can't even recognise that something is off. For instance, if you have regular acne breakouts, but just chalk it up to hormones or your skin type, you may be living with an undiagnosed sensitivity.

Signs of a Food Sensitivity:

- Acne

- Joint pain

- Headaches

- Brain fog

- Bloating

- Diarrhoea

- Gas

- Puffy face

- Eczema

- Dry skin

- Heartburn

If you experience any of these problems on a regular or even semi-regular basis, you may be dealing with a food sensitivity. But don't worry, you are not the only one. It is estimated that 30 million people in the United States alone, have food sensitivities. This is something that we can check and look at for you, through a bioenergetics appointment in my clinic.

Common Foods That Cause Sensitivity

While you could have an intolerance to just about any type of food, there *are* certain foods that more commonly produce problems. Keep in mind this list does not include food allergies—we're simply talking about intolerance and insensitivity here. With the exception of one or two, the foods listed here also cause early ageing. When your body struggles to digest anything, that means your liver, gut, and other internal organs are working overtime to metabolise what are essentially toxins. Remember, your skin is an organ. When your liver isn't able to process those toxins, because it's either too busy working on the overtaxing food items you throw at it, or because your body sees the food itself as a toxin, those toxins start getting released in the only other way your body knows how: through sweat. This is no good for your skin!

- Eggs

- Dairy

- Soy

- Wheat

- Gluten

- Grains

- Sugar

Gluten and refined grains (including sugar) deplete your healthy gut bacteria (which, as we covered, affects your skin health), clog your pores (causing breakouts), and age your skin—whether your system has an intolerance to them or not. But, if you do have a sensitivity to any of these foods, it is likely the problems will be more pronounced or stick around a lot longer.

New research has also pointed to food-related histamine as a trigger for sensitivities, which is created by the fermentation process. So, if the food you're eating contains this, you might be experiencing some symptoms. Some people lack the enzyme to break down histamine, while for others the histamine simply builds up in their system, overloading their gut.

Some examples of histamine foods include:

- Alcoholic beverages

- Anchovies

- Avocados

- Some cheeses

- Cider

- Homemade root beer

- Dried fruits

- Pickles

- Sauerkraut

- Smoked fish

- Sour cream, yoghurt, buttermilk

- Bread with large amounts of yeast

- Vinegar and foods containing large amounts of vinegar

If you suspect that you have a food sensitivity, that doesn't mean you have to eliminate every food I just listed. You do, however, have to start figuring out what foods cause you issues, and make a plan for adjusting your diet accordingly.

Elimination Diet

The tricky part about food sensitivity is that there aren't tests for it at the doctor's surgery like there are for traditional allergies. Instead, it is up to you to connect your symptoms with the food you eat. My team and I can help you do this. Book in a bioenergetics appointment with us, where we can investigate what foods agree with you, and which ones are weakening your body and immune system. You can book an appointment by emailing info@simonethomaswellness.com

To help you connect the dots, I suggest an elimination diet. Going on a short-term elimination diet is often the best and sometimes only way to identify food sensitivities. Often, we may think our upset stomach is caused by one thing, when really it was a hidden product within our food. The only way to find out is by eliminating potential trigger foods and then systematically reintroducing them. You will need at least two months to complete your elimination. The goal is to remove one food at a time, and see if it improves your symptoms. When you are finished, you will have a pretty good picture of what is causing some of these pesky lingering symptoms. Once you understand how your body reacts to certain foods, you can eliminate them entirely from your diet, or just limit how much and how often you eat them. This will really help you to avoid the constant ups and downs of unaddressed food sensitivities.

> You are what you eat.

It's as simple as this for me: when I don't drink enough water or when I eat too much junk food, I can see the right side of my face starting to sag—which I don't like! It makes me feel old. The thing is, it doesn't take years for those changes to manifest; with some foods it can take as little as a weekend of overdoing it for your skin to develop signs such as spots, puffiness, changes in skin tone, premature fine lines and wrinkles, sagging, loss of lustre, or dark circles under the eyes.

Elimination diets can be truly challenging on your own. Cutting out a single food at a time and waiting for one or two months to see a change requires a discipline and commitment that a lot of people may not have, especially with work, kids, friends, family and other commitments all pulling us in different directions. My bioenergetic screenings can accomplish the same thing, all while offering a guide along the way.

I must emphasise that I'm not a GP, but my background is nutrition, weight management, bioenergetics, and hair health. These areas combined give me a solid understanding of how your mind, body, skin and hair work together to form a healthy whole.

Toilet Breaks

This may be the first book you ever read that talks directly about your bathroom habits, but I couldn't leave the skin chapter without mentioning good habits on the toilet! We have talked about how gut health, drinking enough water, and eating the right food all works together to keep your body working properly. Well, the same is true of your bowel movements. How often and how well your body eliminates waste is both a sign of how healthy your system is, and a cause of more problems if it isn't operating properly.

It is important to have a bowel movement every day. Toxins not passed through the bowel actually get rediverted through the skin. As they do so, they cause the utmost damage to collagen and elastin! Poor elimination can be improved by boosting overall gut health, but other ways to improve include drinking more water (as hydration makes stools easier to pass) and including more of the gentler types of fibre in your diet. My Simone Thomas Wellness Super Greens and Everyday Wellbeing are great for encouraging a good exit!

> A moment of sugar on the lips gives extra inches to your hips, and causes fine lines and wrinkles on your face.

Try This

You probably could have guessed what your "Try This" for this chapter was going to be. That's right, it's a food sensitivity elimination log. I'm not going to ask you to cut out all your favourite foods at once, but I am going to ask you to systematically remove each food that has a high likelihood of causing you problems. If you feel brave and have a lot of willpower, then you can eliminate them all at once. BUT—it's important not to cheat! You can't commit to eliminating dairy, without completely eliminating it. Even if you just have it on weekends, then you still won't get a full understanding of what dairy does to your body.

First, use the chart on the next page to analyse the severity and frequency of your symptoms. Next, you will entirely eliminate a food from your diet. You can either do one food at a time or, if you are particularly committed, you can eliminate all the major triggers at once. Either way, you will need to keep them out of your diet for a full month. Once a month has passed, go back to your symptoms list. Take note if each symptom has changed, made progress, or resolved completely.

From there, introduce foods back in one at a time, giving at least two days in between each reintroduction. Again, go back to your chart and take note of how each food reintroduction changes your symptoms, and to what degree.

Elimination Chart

Symptom: Rate the severity and frequency of each symptom from 0-5. (0=you don't experience it, 5=highest severity & frequency)	Elimination Week 1: Reassess the frequency and severity of the symptoms.	Elimination Week 2: Reassess the frequency and severity of the symptoms.	Elimination Week 3: Reassess the frequency and severity of the symptoms.	Elimination Week 4: Reassess the frequency and severity of the symptoms.
Bloating severity: _____ Frequency: _____	Bloating severity: _____ Frequency: _____	Bloating severity: _____ Frequency: _____	Bloating severity: _____ Frequency: _____	Bloating severity: _____ Frequency: _____

Healthy Hair, Happy Body

Gas severity: _____	Gas severity: _____	Gas severity: _____	Gas severity: _____	Gas severity: _____
Frequency: _____	Frequency: _____	Frequency: _____	Frequency: _____	Frequency: _____
Headaches severity: _____	Headaches severity: _____	Headaches severity: _____	Headaches severity: _____	Headaches severity: _____
Frequency: _____	Frequency: _____	Frequency: _____	Frequency: _____	Frequency: _____
Stomach discomfort: _____	Stomach discomfort: _____	Stomach discomfort: _____	Stomach discomfort: _____	Stomach discomfort: _____
Frequency: _____	Frequency: _____	Frequency: _____	Frequency: _____	Frequency: _____

Diarrhoea discomfort: ____ Frequency: ____	Diarrhoea discomfort: ____ Frequency: ____	Diarrhoea discomfort: ____ Frequency: ____	Diarrhoea discomfort: ____ Frequency: ____	Diarrhoea discomfort: ____ Frequency: ____
Breakouts severity: ____ Frequency: ____	Breakouts severity: ____ Frequency: ____	Breakouts severity: ____ Frequency: ____	Breakouts severity: ____ Frequency: ____	Breakouts severity: ____ Frequency: ____
Joint pain severity: ____ Frequency: ____	Joint pain severity: ____ Frequency: ____	Joint pain severity: ____ Frequency: ____	Joint pain severity: ____ Frequency: ____	Joint pain severity: ____ Frequency: ____

Brain fog severity: ———— Frequency: ————	Brain fog severity: ———— Frequency: ————	Brain fog severity: ———— Frequency: ————	Brain fog severity: ———— Frequency: ————	Brain fog severity: ———— Frequency: ————
Heartburn severity: ———— Frequency: ————	Heartburn severity: ———— Frequency: ————	Heartburn severity: ———— Frequency: ————	Heartburn severity: ———— Frequency: ————	Heartburn severity: ———— Frequency: ————
Puffy face severity: ———— Frequency: ————	Puffy face severity: ———— Frequency: ————	Puffy face severity: ———— Frequency: ————	Puffy face severity: ———— Frequency: ————	Puffy face severity: ———— Frequency: ————

Dry skin severity: _____ Frequency: _____	Dry skin severity: _____ Frequency: _____	Dry skin severity: _____ Frequency: _____	Dry skin severity: _____ Frequency: _____	Dry skin severity: _____ Frequency: _____
Other: Severity: _____ Frequency: _____	Other: Severity: _____ Frequency: _____	Other: Severity: _____ Frequency: _____	Other: Severity: _____ Frequency: _____	Other: Severity: _____ Frequency: _____

Reintroduction Chart

Time to do it all over again! As you add foods back in, reassess how you are feeling, noting down each symptom that you experience after two days. Remember, only add one food back in at a time, or else you won't know what caused the symptoms.

Symptom: Rate the severity and frequency of each symptom from 0-5. (0=you don't experience it, 5=highest severity & frequency)	Food One: Reassess the frequency and severity of the symptoms.	Food Two: Reassess the frequency and severity of the symptoms.	Food Three: Reassess the frequency and severity of the symptoms.	Food Four: Reassess the frequency and severity of the symptoms.

Bloating severity: _____ Frequency: _____	Bloating severity: _____ Frequency: _____	Bloating severity: _____ Frequency: _____	Bloating severity: _____ Frequency: _____	Bloating severity: _____ Frequency: _____
Gas severity: _____ Frequency: _____	Gas severity: _____ Frequency: _____	Gas severity: _____ Frequency: _____	Gas severity: _____ Frequency: _____	Gas severity: _____ Frequency: _____
Headaches severity: _____ Frequency: _____	Headaches severity: _____ Frequency: _____	Headaches severity: _____ Frequency: _____	Headaches severity: _____ Frequency: _____	Headaches severity: _____ Frequency: _____

Stomach discomfort: _____ Frequency: _____	Stomach discomfort: _____ Frequency: _____	Stomach discomfort: _____ Frequency: _____	Stomach discomfort: _____ Frequency: _____	Stomach discomfort: _____ Frequency: _____
Diarrhoea discomfort: _____ Frequency: _____	Diarrhoea discomfort: _____ Frequency: _____	Diarrhoea discomfort: _____ Frequency: _____	Diarrhoea discomfort: _____ Frequency: _____	Diarrhoea discomfort: _____ Frequency: _____
Breakouts severity: _____ Frequency: _____	Breakouts severity: _____ Frequency: _____	Breakouts severity: _____ Frequency: _____	Breakouts severity: _____ Frequency: _____	Breakouts severity: _____ Frequency: _____

Joint pain severity: _____ Frequency: _____	Joint pain severity: _____ Frequency: _____	Joint pain severity: _____ Frequency: _____	Joint pain severity: _____ Frequency: _____	Joint pain severity: _____ Frequency: _____
Brain fog severity: _____ Frequency: _____	Brain fog severity: _____ Frequency: _____	Brain fog severity: _____ Frequency: _____	Brain fog severity: _____ Frequency: _____	Brain fog severity: _____ Frequency: _____
Heartburn severity: _____ Frequency: _____	Heartburn severity: _____ Frequency: _____	Heartburn severity: _____ Frequency: _____	Heartburn severity: _____ Frequency: _____	Heartburn severity: _____ Frequency: _____

Puffy face severity: ____ Frequency: ____	Puffy face severity: ____ Frequency: ____	Puffy face severity: ____ Frequency: ____	Puffy face severity: ____ Frequency: ____	Puffy face severity: ____ Frequency: ____
Dry skin severity: ____ Frequency: ____	Dry skin severity: ____ Frequency: ____	Dry skin severity: ____ Frequency: ____	Dry skin severity: ____ Frequency: ____	Dry skin severity: ____ Frequency: ____
Other: Severity: ____ Frequency: ____	Other: Severity: ____ Frequency: ____	Other: Severity: ____ Frequency: ____	Other: Severity: ____ Frequency: ____	Other: Severity: ____ Frequency: ____

Chapter Eleven: Products and Care

I could write an entire book on the dos and don'ts of skin and hair care products that flood the market. But, since I only have a chapter, I will keep it to the basics. It is up to you to do your homework on the products you are using. Rule number one—don't fall for gimmicks. Facebook and YouTube ads are especially tempting, because they are expertly formulated to trigger your insecurities, hopes, and fears. Facebook, YouTube, and Google all have ways of knowing what you are searching for on your computer, so if you have been looking for "ways to grow your hair" or "how to make my skin softer" they are seeing that and marketing every possible related product. That doesn't mean, however, that the products you are seeing have been vetted, that they actually work, or that they are safe.

So, how do you find products that actually do work? I follow a few simple rules when purchasing new products:

Simone's Rules for Products

1. **Short ingredients list**. Just like you want your food to have as few ingredients as possible, the same rule applies to products you are using. This limits the possibility of additives, preservatives, and weird chemicals that will both irritate your skin and cause more harm than good in the long run.

2. **No soaps, detergents, or alcohol**. All of these things are way too harsh and completely unnecessary for our skin. Your skin is pretty

good at taking care of itself. When we use harsh soaps, detergents, or alcohol, we are stripping our skin of its natural oils, causing an imbalance and preventing its natural immune systems from working.

3. **No paraben or sulphates**. Both paraben and sulphates are preservatives. These are meant to keep your products fresh, and deter bacterial growth. Parabens have been linked to breast cancer; in lab studies when parabens are introduced to cancer cells, the cancer grows faster. The dangers of sulphates can be less severe, but if you have a sensitivity to them then they have been known to cause hypotension, abdominal pain, dermatitis, and even in some rare cases, anaphylaxis. Your best (and safest) bet is to stay away from them altogether.

4. **Stick with natural products**. This means products not made with chemicals. Most of what your skin and hair needs can be found directly in nature, like aloe, chamomile, vitamin C, and rosewater. The list goes on and on. Why use synthetic products meant to replicate something that nature does better, and without extra side-effects too?

5. **Be wary of scents**. If you have sensitive skin, products with aggressive scents might cause irritation. And, truthfully, they aren't necessary. Look for natural, light scents (if that's something you enjoy) or find your scents elsewhere (candles or perfumes) so you don't have to apply them directly to the skin.

6. **Choose personalised and targeted products**. The products you choose should be specific to your skin or hair type. There are certainly different products for curly hair, coarse hair, or fine/thin hair, and it's the same with your skin products. If your skin is dry, don't use products designed for oily skin! Know your skin and hair, and find products that cater to you.

7. **Use cream-based cleansers and moisturisers for your face**. Cream cleansers provide an extra boost of moisture while they cleanse. Gel cleansers and moisturisers can unnecessarily dry out your skin.

8. **Download the "Think Dirty" app**. This app makes it easy to figure out exactly what you are slathering onto your face, lips, body, and hair. Simply use the app to take a picture of your product, and they will tell you all the nasty things that you probably want to avoid.

9. **Investing in good products.** As we do with our food, it is important to invest in good products for our skin and hair. If you aren't sure, then treat yourself to an afternoon at one of the many product counters across a number of department stores. Get yourself familiar with the products and see what you feel works best with your skin and hair. Look for organic products, not tested on animals, that come from a natural background rather than being chemically produced.

Skin Care Guide

Once again, I find that I could write an entire book on how to take care of your skin, but instead I will lay down the basics for you. Unlike your hair, which goes through cycles, your skin is constantly re-growing cells without a break. So, it is extra important to take the time each day to care for your skin properly. I would suggest setting yourself up with a routine. Like anything that may be new, it is a good idea to make a plan and set up a schedule. Otherwise, it's unrealistic to incorporate all or any of my suggestions.

- **Try a tinted moisturiser.** Tinted moisturiser is a great way to provide a little colour without having to cover up your natural glow with makeup. In fact, I very rarely wear foundation unless it's to an awards ceremony or photographic shoot. Day to day I love my skin and like to see my natural glow.

- **Wash your face twice a day**, and **never sleep in your makeup**. Makeup doesn't have a lot of documented adverse effects, as long as you take it off each day. Sleeping in your makeup can have some nasty adverse consequences, like clogged pores, breakouts, inflammation, rash, premature ageing, and in some cases can cause infection.

- **Wash your makeup brushes.** If you use makeup brushes, it's incredibly important to give them a thorough cleaning every week or so. You may have the best routine for your face and skin, but if you aren't cleaning your brushes then the bacteria that you are washing off your face is simply growing on your brushes.

- **Treat yourself to a really rich night cream.** During the day, you should be using a lighter moisturiser for your face that contains some level of SPF. Even in the winter, you want to protect your skin from the harmful effects of the sun. Night, however, is a different story. While daytime moisturisers protect your skin, night moisturisers do the heavy lifting with correcting. At night, your skin is better at absorbing active ingredients and nutrients, so you want to choose a night cream that fits your skin profile.

- **Moisturise your body.** Most of us, hopefully, have a habit of moisturising our face each day after we wash, but it is just as important to moisturise your body. Unlike your face care routine, there is no set frequency to which you should moisturise. Instead, listen to your body. Moisturise as often as your skin needs it. For some people that might mean every day. For others, it is once every other day or only a few times a week. I love good old Palmer's Coconut Lotion; I have used this for years.

- **Moisturise your feet and hands.** It's easy to neglect these extremities when we are working through our skincare routine, but they are just as important, if not more so. Our hands and feet often show more signs of damage, age, and dryness because of excessive washing and the rigours we put them through every day. Some dermatologists have even suggested moisturising the hands after every wash. That may be too impractical for you, but you should moisturise at least once a day. Again, I use Palmer's for this.

- **Use a face mask.** First and foremost, facial masks are a great way to pamper yourself and get a little downtime, without the added expense of a full price facial at the beauty salon. But facemasks have the added benefit of packing in a lot of skin firming and replenishing nutrients into one little mask. Leaving a nutrient-rich mask on your skin for fifteen to twenty minutes means you give it a chance to really absorb. Typically, we wash our face first, then apply the mask, so the daily build-up doesn't get in the way of absorption. There are many varying types of masks, each targeted for different problems or types of skin. A charcoal mask purifies, while an aloe mask calms, with countless others in between. The latest craze is sheet masks that come in single-use packages, in which you apply the sheet directly to your face. The theory is that with the contact of the sheet, the products absorb better. Regardless of the mask you choose, using one on a regular basis gives your skin an extra boost.

- **Exfoliate.** The goal of exfoliating the skin is to remove dead skin cells, pollution, environmental toxins, accelerate cellular renewal, and encourage collagen production. Look for an exfoliant that doesn't contain large particles. The exfoliant should be fine, like tiny grains of sand, otherwise you risk doing more damage than good. The jury is still out on how often you should exfoliate your skin. Read the label on your exfoliant for how often it is intended to be used. Most people aim for twice a week.

- **Epsom/Lavender Bath.** You may be one of those people who has a misconception about the purpose and benefits of a nightly soak in the bath, thinking it is only for toddlers and older ladies, but there are many health benefits for your whole body and your skin. An Epsom or lavender bath soak helps relieve stress, relieves aches and pains, helps muscles and nerves function properly, and helps eliminate toxins from the body—all of which helps your skin have a healthy glow.

- **Change your pillowcase.** This may just seem like common sense hygiene, but you should be changing your pillowcase regularly. And just as importantly, you should toss those old cotton pillowcases and opt instead for silk. Silk pillowcases don't steal your skin (and your hair's) moisture while you sleep. Silk also has a nice cooling effect, which makes sleep more comfortable as an added bonus.

- **Have a facial on a regular basis.** If you have never had a facial, then you don't know what you're missing! A facial is a great way to get some self-care in while also taking care of your skin. Facials can stimulate collagen production, eliminate toxins in your skin, boost circulation to the skin, and provide a deep-clean and intensive moisturiser.

- **Don't forget your supplements!** To keep the elasticity in your skin, try my Wellness "SkinQuencher" tablets, bursting with type I marine collagen and vitamin C. I like to take mine at night to help with the immune system, or thirty minutes before a heavy workout, because it really does make a difference.

- **Say no to sunbeds.** Despite all of the research to prove how dangerous artificial sunbeds are, many people are still using them. Why not walk to work and get your daily fix of sunlight? Or park twenty minutes away, as I do, for exercise and to clear my head before and after work. You can use that time to get your extra boost of vitamins. Even in the winter or on cloudy days, you will still get the benefits.

Hair Care Guide

Unfortunately, there is no single, one-size-fits-all hair care guide. The advice I give to someone with thinning, straight hair would be entirely different to someone with thick curly hair. We describe hair with various different adjectives: thick, curly, thin, wavy. All of these things are in large part determined by genetics, but understanding your hair type will help you to take better care of it. We will go over five defining factors for your hair before getting into how best to take care of it, factoring in porosity, diameter, density, curl pattern, and elasticity.

Porosity

Porosity refers to how well your hair absorbs moisture and chemicals. Most people know if their hair is highly porous (even if they never knew the word for it) because their hair reacts quickly to humidity and always seems dry, no matter how much moisturising conditioner they use. On the other hand, low porosity hair can be just as hard to moisturise, because nothing is being absorbed and it doesn't react to humidity. If you suspect that your hair is highly porous, you may want to try a moisture-sealing process that starts with a water-based moisturising product followed by an oil-based product, which acts as a barrier from moisture loss. If you have low porosity hair, focus on a conditioner with a pH value of 4.5-5.5. Be aware, if your hair is porous then it probably has sustained some damage that has stripped it of its natural defences.

Texture

It is pretty easy to tell what texture your hair is. While some people have a mix, most people fall into three categories: curly, straight, or wavy. Major changes in hormones, including puberty, pregnancy, menopause, and childbirth can also change the texture of your hair.

Straight

Straight hair is often sleek and shiny, but can quickly become greasy and limp. It can be thick or thin and is often reluctant to hold a curl. Typically, when caring for and styling straight hair, it's important to keep it clean to prevent that greasy, limp look. We also want to avoid cuticle damage by gently brushing the hair and limiting heated styling.

Wavy

Wavy hair is right in the middle of curly and straight hair. Waves can be soft, subtle, or have more definition. Focus on your styling techniques to emphasise the natural pattern of your hair and prevent tangling.

Curly

Curls come in a wide variety, from loose curls to spirals and tight cork-screws. Regardless of your type, curls often need more care than other types of hair, especially since they tend toward the drier side. Hydrating masks and conditioning treatments are essential to keep the "frizz" down.

Elasticity

The elasticity of your hair refers to how easily it breaks under pressure. Hair that has high elasticity is healthy hair. On the other hand, low elasticity means your hair is probably too dry, damaged, and unhealthy. You need to be extra cautious when doing chemical treatments to your hair and when choosing your hair products. Gauge elasticity with one to four strands of wet hair. When you pull at opposite ends and let go, your hair should be able to stretch about 50% of its length and still go back to its original shape. If your hair is damaged, it will only stretch about 20% before breaking.

Diameter

Diameter is the thickness of each individual hair strand. We determine diameter by comparing a strand of hair to sewing thread. If your hair is thinner than the thread, you have a small diameter. Conversely, if it's bigger than the thread, you have high diameter, and if it is the same size, you have normal diameter. Your hair's diameter is a factor in elasticity. If you've lost hair, it may grow back with a smaller diameter, but should with time and care return to normal. Understanding the diameter of the hair helps us better find the right products. If your hair is fine (small diameter) then you need lightweight products, while larger diameters require heavier products. Products that claim to make your hair thicker are either using a very low or high pH to make the hair swell, or they are using polymers that affix to the hair, to give it a temporary added thickness.

Density

Density refers to how many follicles you have per square inch. Find this by pulling your hair back into a ponytail. If the ponytail is about the size of a five-pence piece, you have low hair density. If it is the size of a ten-pence piece, then you have medium density, and if it is the size of a fifty-pence piece then you have high density. Much like diameter, you can't really change the density of your hair, but understanding your hair density helps you monitor the health of your hair. If your density decreases, you know something is wrong.

Advice for All Hair Types

- **Say no to sulphates.** In the past, most shampoos used sulphates, originally designed to remove engine oil. After we realised that these were simply too harsh for hair, more variety came onto the market, using humectants, fatty acids, and emollients. My favourite brand that I use on clients, and which I highly recommend, is Davines. Check them out online!

- **Find a moisturising mask.** Once-a-week moisturising masks do exactly as the name suggests—adding back nourishing moisture that your hair needs.

- **Take it easy on the heat.** I understand that using hairdryers, curling irons, and straighteners all help to get that perfect night-on-the-town look, but try not to overheat your hair, as that can cause over-drying, damage, and breaking.

- **Schedule regular haircuts.** A good haircut can have a huge impact on the appearance, shape, and feel of your hair, but it can also help prevent further damage. If your hair has split ends, then this means that the oldest parts of your hair have become damaged and split apart. The only way to remove split ends is by cutting them. If you don't remove them regularly, the split will continue up the shaft of the hair until the entire strand is damaged. Don't believe those products that claim they can heal a split end. They may temporarily give the appearance of healed splits through the use of polymers, but the hair is still split regardless. Sometimes a fresh haircut is the new start your hair needs.

- **Avoid harsh chemicals.** Harsh chemicals that are meant to straighten, curl, or colour your hair, essentially change the chemical composition of your hair. When they do this, they break down its natural defences, sometimes permanently. These chemical treatments—such as perms and relaxers—are designed to break the bonds of your hair and reform them. This makes your hair weaker with each treatment.

- **Keep it natural.** This piece of advice should come as no surprise given the "all-natural" trend through the rest of this book, but too many people don't consider the chemicals and additives in their hair care products. They think that because they're just putting it on their hair, it won't make a difference to the rest of their body. I am here to say, it does make a difference. Toxins in your hair affect your scalp health and your skin health too. The beauty industry is notorious for loading up their products with questionable ingredients. So, apply the same rules for haircare to foods and skincare. The fewer ingredients, the better. Stick with natural ingredients and avoid toxins such as parabens, artificial fragrances, triclosan, and polyethylene glycol (PEG).

Try This

Take a look at the hair and skin products you have in your bathroom. Then, clean them out! In the same way that we cleaned our cupboards of all the unhealthy, counterproductive foods that would set back our clean lifestyle, we need to do the same with our hair and skin products. Some of us may have products that expired two years ago, just living in the back of our bathroom cupboard. Others probably have at least one or two products that fall into my "no-no" category, but you won't know until you start casting a critical eye across each one. If you come across products that don't serve your goals right now, then they belong in the bin. I don't care if it was your favourite lip gloss in middle school, or if one time you got a compliment on the scent of your shampoo—it's time to cut those old unhealthy ties and make room for your new healthy hair and skin lifestyle!

Chapter Twelve: Making It Your Own

Here we are, at the end of all the advice I could cram into this one little primer. I hope that throughout this book you have taken the time to complete each "Try This". Each one was designed to give you a solid foundation and understanding of each lifestyle change. Now, it's up to you to decide where you go next. If most of the information in this book was brand new to you, then you might want to stick closely to the "Try This" diets, plans and tips. However, when you start to feel more comfortable, you can start making healthy, clean lifestyle changes in your own, individual way.

As I said at the beginning of this book, the journey toward a healthier lifestyle and all the benefits it can provide will be unique to you. What works for one person doesn't always work for another. This book stemmed from people who have hair and scalp issues, but all of it has an impact on our lifestyles, health, and living healthier. The whole point of this journey was hair growth, reduced hair loss, reduced scalp inflammation, improved skin conditions, and reduced fatigue. If you started reading this book for a narrow purpose, you may have started noticing other benefits as well, like having more energy and better sleep patterns.

As a nutrition coach, it has always been my aim to dispel the myth that poor hair and skin health occurs "just because". There is a reason, and there is a solution, and it normally starts with what you're putting onto your skin and hair, and into your body (and in some cases what is inside your body or what is not inside, meaning what you are lacking). Consumers have become conditioned to use poor quality products, simply because of well-present-ed adverts on TV, or fancy packaging. But, it doesn't have to be this way. Above all things, this book should have given you awareness: awareness that the products you're using have an enormous impact on your health, and awareness that **it is** possible to break negative health cycles. And, breaking those cycles can be a wonderful, exciting, and fun experience!

Remember, it doesn't have to be a mountain, and it certainly shouldn't feel that way either. With the help of Simone Thomas Wellness, you can make the transition enjoyable. You'll know from my own personal story that clean living has made me feel empowered, so much so that I've made a career from empowering others to do the same. There is incredible joy to be had in taking back control of your health, in purging your cupboards and home of toxic products. These products are deliberately designed to trap you in a harmful cycle. You've been led to believe that you need them, but you don't! All you need is the courage and self-belief to acknowledge your own worth, to recognise that you can reclaim your body, right now!

You have the power to change your health, and I have the knowledge and expertise to help you make this a reality. So, let's get together and start the ball rolling. We're all partners on this clean living journey, and I can't wait to meet each and every one of you.

Simone Thomas.

The New Alphabet

With the help of some of my clients, we came up with a new alphabet to keep you on track and remind you of the most important pieces in your new and improved lifestyle. On some, I couldn't resist giving them a double meaning, because there is just too much for only twenty-six!

A is for APPLE. One a day will certainly help you keep that doctor away! Always make sure that your fruit and vegetables are ORGANIC when possible.

B is for BREATHE. More deeply, more soundly, more often.

C is for CARE. For yourself, my darlings, take at least fifteen minutes a day to just sit and do what you want to do. It's amazing how a feeling of self-worth increases your wellbeing. Also, care for your cosmetics. Every day we coat our faces in makeup. We use ten to thirty products a day on our bodies, whether that is simple skincare or makeup. In the end, that exposes us to toxins and carcinogenic ingredients. Always check labels and stick to organic products.

D is for DRINK all day. Just flush that glorious system through. Drink a minimum of eight glasses a day, and believe me your skin and mind will reflect the glowing results.

E is for ENJOY. Take time to enjoy your food; turn off your phone or any digital device and look at your plate of food while eating. Chew each mouthful thoroughly before swallowing.

F is for FEAR OF MISSING OUT. The average person spends over 2 hours on their phone each day! Time yourself. Check your phone 4 times daily only, and narrow it down to 4 sessions of 15 minutes. Once you've achieved this, you've already halved it! You'll be amazed at how quickly this time goes, and it will seriously make you think about how long you used to spend on it in the first place.

G is for GLUTEN FREE. It's amazing how much better I felt when I omitted gluten from my diet. It's also incredible how many people are in some way gluten intolerant and don't know it.

H is for HAPPY. If you're happy and you know it clap your hands—if you're not, then let's do something about it!

I is for IDEA. If you have an idea that has always been at the back of your mind on the list of "oh, I'd love to do that", start paving the way little by little to make it happen, so you are ready for the day that you do.

J is for JANUARY. This always used to be the month that you started your diet. Well, you won't ever have to welcome January with dread again, as you aren't on a diet and never will be. You've simply changed your eating habits!

K is for KISS. Make sure you kiss the ones you love the most at least once a day. You'll be amazed at just how many kisses you get back!

L is for LOVE THYSELF. No, you're not being selfish, but if you want to book a manicure, facial, or pedicure then go ahead—it's called maintenance. As I write this, I am away for a week of self-love at Homefield Grange—the most amazing retreat. This is a must-do for those who want to check in on themselves, and give their mind and body something back.

M is for MAINTENANCE. Only you will have the privilege of knowing your body all your life. So, look after it. Ensure the fuel you choose is premium, and that your water and oil levels are monitored daily. M is also for metabolism—every day our bodies make toxins. As our stress increases, our toxins increase. Keep an eye on your metabolism to keep those toxins in check.

N is for NEW YOU. You will seriously start seeing a new you in less than 3 months. Strangely enough, with your hair and skin looking amazing, your body will too. If you abide by the Saints and not the Sinners, weight will naturally drop. And, most importantly, it will stay off.

O is for ORGASM. The best stress release ever is an amazing, earth-shattering orgasm; you can feel the stress and strains leave your body immediately. Ensure that you enjoy a daily orgasm, and if you need a little help in that department then there are tools available to achieve this. O also stands for organic. Our foods can be riddled with antibiotics, hormones, pesticides and artificial preservatives, colourants, and flavours. When you can, always go organic, even for children. Cook fresh, avoid sugar, and don't over salt.

P is for PACKED LUNCH. Learn to do it regularly! Always cook too much meat or fish for dinner, and pop it into a chilled container (along with some salad and fruit) for the next day's lunch.

Q is for QUEER EYE for a STRAIGHT GAL. It's "guy" actually, but oh I do so love that series! It's amazing how a new look completely transforms a person's confidence. Ask your best gay friend how he thinks you look. Take him shopping with you and let him cull your wardrobe.

R is for REVIVE. Yes, we all get burnout, so find that quiet, calm place—whether it's a day spa or a triple viewing at the cinema. You've earned it.

S is for SPEAKERPHONE. Use the speakerphone whenever you can. This will protect your brain from the radiation emitted from your mobile phone. Be a SWAN—when you are bent over your digital device, the pressure on your neck is equivalent to 60 pounds. Keep your neck long, and you will soon notice the difference.

T is for TECHNOLOGY. We need to be in control of our relationship with technology, and not the other way around.

U is for U. Look after it!

V is for VICE VERSA. We work, we have families, people need to communicate with us and vice-versa. Aim to be plugged in whilst digitally detoxing.

W is for WALK. Walk outdoors, and do it often. But also, water Water is so key. Always choose filtered water, and invest in a water filter for home or buy a bottle that can filter it for you. Unfiltered water contains agricultural and pharmaceutical waste, as well as chlorine, heavy metals, and pesticides.

X is for KISS and MAKE UP before bedtime.

Y is for YOUNG. It's all about thinking, saying, talking, and staying YOUNG.

Z is for ZZZZ. Get a good night's sleep. Go to bed when you are tired; don't fight it and you will wake up happy!

LOOK WHAT YOU MADE ME DO!

I wanted to leave you with some real stories of success from clients who have followed my program and changed their lives. Each of these stories represents the hard work, dedication, and trust of individuals who sought me out for a variety of reasons. Many of them came to me as a last resort after struggling with hair loss, poor health, and skin issues for most of their lives. Others just hoped I could provide some insight into what was happening with their bodies. Regardless of their reasons for seeking me out, in the end they discovered habits that changed their lives, and you can too!

Road of Discovery and Healing, Teagan

I met Simone when she first opened her salon in Westbourne. I had the pleasure of interviewing Simone for a local magazine, and I was in awe at everything she had achieved and her goals for the future. What's crazy is that Simone has now achieved *all* of those goals that she told me about in that interview! As a hair-extension lover, I was in my dream shop when walking into Simone's salon. We soon became friends, which all began over our love of hair ☺. Simone then went on to open Simone Thomas Salon, which became my firm favourite salon to attend if my hair needed a bit of TLC.

It was in 2018 when I was straightening my hair, that I saw a thin patch on the side of my head. When I looked on the other side, I had a matching patch there too. As someone who doesn't really like getting my hair cut because I want long locks, I went into complete panic mode. I messaged Simone, as I knew she was the expert in this, and she asked me to come over to check out my hair.

When I arrived, Simone looked over my hair, and asked me a lot of questions about my hair, health, and habits to try and understand what was going on. Simone concluded it was my use of clip-in hair extensions that had over the years pulled on my hair roots. She assured me it would grow back with some extra TLC. She told me about a scalp microdermabrasion at Simone Thomas Salon that would be great to stimulate my hair follicles, advising me on what shampoos, conditioners and brushes to use, and explaining how important it was to blow dry my hair every time I washed it—to make sure there was no dampness left on my scalp.

During my nutrition and bioenergetics consultation, it came to light that Simone thought I had a condition called endometritis. After speaking to her, I agreed to go for a consultation with a doctor, where I learned that Simone was correct—I did have endometritis, which required surgery to remove. Just one year later, my hair grew back, thanks to Simone's incredible advice. Simone supported me through the entire process with continuous and regular check-ins and advice. She is an absolute walking angel, and

Healthy Hair, Happy Body

I couldn't thank her more for all the help and support she has given to me, that has not only helped my hair but also my health too. I am very lucky to be able to call Simone a dear friend of mine.

I have just started Simone's wellness products, and I am already feeling healthier and happier. I am so excited to continue with these products and see what the real change is for me. Also, I am now currently seven months pregnant—something which I never thought would be possible!

Cure for Fatigue and Malaise, Sarah

I have just started taking Simone Thomas Wellness Supplements, and I am already feeling healthier and happier. I am so excited to continue with these products and see what the real change is for me. Before I started following Simone's programme, I felt lethargic and tired all the time. My hair would fall out every time I washed it, which was daily, because I was prone to greasy hair. My skin, for my age, was pretty good aside from the dark circles under my eyes, which I blamed on near-constant exhaustion. Despite always being tired, sleep never came easily. Some nights I wouldn't drift off until 2:00-3:00 a.m. I suffered from hot flushes so badly that my entire body would feel sweaty and clammy. And, if that wasn't bad enough, I lived with nearly constant urine infections.

When I started to take Simone Thomas Wellness Gingko plan, I couldn't believe it. WOW, how different I felt! I had more energy and my body felt more alive. I couldn't believe how much my hair grew and how thick it was. I was actually witnessing new hair growth! It looked so much thicker and fuller—what's more, I wasn't losing it! Everybody noticed the difference (even my husband!). I also found I could wash my hair every other day. My skin, that I never thought was too bad, showed improvements too, as my dark circles diminished. Although my urine infections didn't stop, they didn't happen as often as they used to, with just two in the entire three-month course. My hot flushes calmed, and I was always fast asleep around midnight. I started to find I was attracted to eating healthier foods too.

Whilst taking these tablets, I felt better than I had in a long time. Simone's treatment has totally changed my life, and I'm so grateful and happy that we went on this journey together.

Chance Meeting Leads to Inner and Outer Healing, Kelly

I am fortunate enough to have met Simone through her son, Ashton. I can remember meeting Simone before her son started at the school where I work. Simone was like a "ray of sunshine", I thought, and she radiated all around her. NOT at all like the typical "I LOVE ME, WHO DO YOU LOVE?" women you meet or see on the telly!!!

Healthy Hair, Happy Body

Simone has a passion for life; for her life and others. You cannot help but let down all your own personal barriers, telling her all your woes. Somehow that is exactly what I did.

My colleague and I were fortunate enough to have some hair products from Simone, and these alone blew us away! Not sure my hair knew what had hit it, and I thought it could not look any better. Having then chatted with Simone about the hair products, we just got talking. For the first time in a very long time, I opened up about all that I had gone through. Albeit a shortened version, but that was enough for Simone to make me feel the way I do today, and I will NEVER be able to thank her enough.

Thirteen years ago, we lost our son, Sam, and I was put on anti-depressants. Since then I've never had an appointment with the doctors to check how I am nor to see if I wanted to come off them. Being in a rather odd place mentally, overweight, tired, anxious, VERY low libido, nervous, and on these tablets, I visited Simone, who gave me her range of "Simone Thomas Wellness" supplements.

Well...

I can honestly say, once you get over the smell of the toxins leaving your body, I FELT FANTASTIC!!!!!!!!! WHERE HAVE YOU BEEN ALL OUR LIVES SIMONE THOMAS!!!!!

Everyone I meet has commented on my skin and how well I look, which for me is a huge compliment in itself, as I have had 2 moles removed, which left scars that I am self-conscious about. These, may I add, look smoother and softer all the time! My hair is thicker and shinier and seems to last so much longer between washes too. Simone advised me to stop following the slimming world diet to a degree, as lots of their meal plans are full of nasties and can take years to leave the body. She advised me to just keep to a diet of fresh ingredients and only from the land, sea, and tree/bush. Although chocolate and crisps, my downfall, are NOT in these categories, the weight is falling off me. I no longer feel sluggish, but lighter and cleaner. I no longer feel tired, but full of energy and have even started to use the gym member-ship that I had been paying for over the past 2 years!! GOODBYE anxiety, GOODBYE negative thoughts, and HELLO to someone that I didn't know I was capable of being.

Look out world...if you want to feel fantastic, have a real desire in life again, and above all want to do this for YOU, then listen to what Simone has to say. Believe in what she says. Trust me, you will not be disappointed. I could shout from the rooftops—I want the world to know about these products and cannot help but tell everyone I meet about them. Purely because my face and hair say it all. I am smiling, I am shining from the inside and out, and I will be forever grateful to you, Simone. Thank you will never be enough.

Healthy Hair, Happy Body

Sticking to a Plan and Getting Happy, Sharelle

I am so happy with my results so far, and look forward to more changes in my mind and body. I have been on the Biotin plan and SkinQuencher supplements to resolve my acne for the past four months. I suffer from Polycystic Ovary Syndrome (PCOS), and after not receiving the help I needed from professionals, I asked Simone for help with my hair and general wellbeing. She gave me advice on nutritious foods that my body needed, to help with PCOS, as well as foods to avoid and exercises I can do daily to target my problem areas. Since starting this plan, I have lost weight, my skin became so much clearer, my hormones started to balance out, and my hair feels and looks amazing as well. Even my boyfriend has noticed changes in me. Before I met Simone, I was so unhappy and depressed, but now I am thriving and looking forward to a happier, healthier future.

Now it's time to make your own inspirational story. Find your truth, your passion, your health, and your commitment, and start on the path of health and healing!

Trading Post

Abel and Cole https://www.abelandcole.co.uk/

Almond Cow https://almondcow.co/

Barbara Cox https://www.barbaracox.mc/

Brooke Burke https://brookeburke.com/

Calm App https://www.calm.com/

Coconut Collaborative https://coconutco.co.uk/

Courtney Black https://www.courtneyblack.co.uk/

Daily Yoga App https://dailyyoga.com/

Davines https://www.davines.com/

Homefield Grange https://www.homefieldgrangeretreat.co.uk/

Lucy Bee https://lucybee.com/

Palmers Coconut Lotion https://uk.palmers.com/

Peloton https://www.onepeloton.co.uk/

The Power of Habit, Charles Duhigg https://charlesduhigg.com/the-power-of-habit/

Tisserand Aroma Spa https://www.tisserand.com/

Waitrose https://www.waitrose.com/